Young, female and black

CLITBEC

Young black women symbolise the effects of the inequalities of British society. They do well at school and are good, efficient workers, yet as a group they consistently fail to secure the economic status and occupational prestige of their white counterparts.

Heidi Safia Mirza, a black woman sociologist, charts the experience of a group of young black women as they leave school and enter the world of work, and investigates why black women suffer these injustices. She challenges the widely-held myth that young black women underachieve both at school and in the labour market, and provides evidence that goes beyond current notions of black female identity. She reveals the processes of inequality that, despite meritocratic ideals, persist in western society, shifting the emphasis from an analysis of identity towards an examination of the central role of the social and economic disadvantage in the education system.

Through a comparative study of research and writing from America, Britain and the Caribbean, *Young, Female and Black* re-examines our present understanding of what is meant by educational underachievement, the black family and, in particular, black womanhood in Britain. A forceful and positive reappraisal of the experience of black women, it will be essential reading for students of sociology, education, social policy, race relations and feminist thought.

Young, female and black

Heidi Safia Mirza

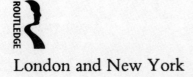

London and New York

First published in 1992
by Routledge
11 New Fetter Lane, London EC4P 4EE

Simultaneously published in the USA and Canada
by Routledge
a division of Routledge, Chapman and Hall, Inc.
29 West 35th Street, New York, NY 10001

© 1992 Heidi Safia Mirza

Typeset by LaserScript, Mitcham, Surrey
Printed and bound in Great Britain by Clays Ltd, St Ives plc

British Library Cataloguing in Publication Data

Mirza, Heidi Safia
    Young, female and black.
    I. Title
    305.48896

Library of Congress Cataloging in Publication Data

Mirza, Heidi Safia, 1958–
    Young, female and black/Heidi Safia Mirza.
    p.   cm.
    Includes bibliographical references and index.
    1. Women, Black – Great Britain – Social conditions. 2. Great
    Britain – Race relations. I. Title.
    DA125.N4M57   1992
    305.48′896041–dc20   91-30180

ISBN 0–415–06704–9
      0–415–06705-7 (pbk)

For Aliya

Contents

Acknowledgements

I was inspired to undertake this project on young black women by Professor Alan Little, who will always be fondly remembered.

I am also indebted to Dr John Stone who has been a very special colleague: patient, encouraging and resourceful; and to Tunde Oluwa without whose strength and support I could not have completed this book.

To my special friends Nasim Govanni, June Williams and Stewart Phillips, who contributed each in their own way.

To the teachers, parents and young people who took part in the study, willingly sharing their experiences and giving me their time. In the text their names are fictional.

A special 'thank you' to Hilary Cox, Greg Fegan and Iris Swain for their technical and computing expertise.

I would like to express my thanks and appreciation to Thelma and Camran Mirza for their special help.

Finally, to my mother, father and brother, Hilda, Ralph and Gerard Hosier, and in particular my daughter, Aliya, whose love and consideration have been a tower of strength.

Chapter 1

Introduction

Universal education – that is, compulsory, free schooling for all – is an essential and valued aspect of liberal democratic society. Its promise of social mobility through the acquisition of academic credentials offers each individual, regardless of social origin, the dream of equality. However, in spite of this meritocratic ideal, inequality among certain groups has remained endemic. One such group is African Caribbean women. This book, an investigation into the factors that influence the job choices of young black female school leavers, is an attempt to understand the process of inequality which so clearly structures their lives.

In the late seventies the work of the cultural reproductionists dominated the analysis of social inequality in Britain. During this time Paul Willis, an influential scholar within this tradition, asked the question, 'How is it that working-class kids come to get working-class jobs?' His answer was very perceptive; he put forward the notion of the 'counter-school culture'. The counter-school culture was a culture of resistance to school and the authority it imposes. Willis suggested that young white men, through their own activity and ideological development, reproduce themselves as a working class. It was a radical and challenging observation.

In the eighties the notion of 'subcultures of resistance', the legacy of the cultural reproductionist school of thought, became the perceived wisdom for not only explaining the persistence of working-class inequality, but also sexual and racial inequality. But what if some 'kids' identify with school, do relatively well, but still fail to attain the jobs they have aspired to? If such an anomaly exists it calls into question the operation of the counter-school culture and other cultures of resistance.

However, it is exactly this phenomenon, positive educational orientation in the context of persistent labour-market inequality, that is the collective experience of young black British women. Despite this contrary evidence, subcultural analysis has become, and remains, the major influence on the small but distinct body of scholarship which examines the experiences of young black women in Britain.

This preoccupation with subculture has had far-reaching consequences for the study of black women in Britain. Romantic notions of black female subcultures of resistance prevail in both our commonsense and academic discussions. At the core of these representations has been the belief that black females are motivated primarily through identification with their 'strong black mothers'. The matriarchal family structure, in which motherhood takes on a special meaning, is seen as a resource. It is implied that the maternal role model provides black women with special powers of endurance which especially equip them in their struggle against racism and sexism at home, in school and the work place.

While black women clearly do have strong cultural traditions that are historically distinct, such a celebratory emphasis is analytically naïve for several reasons. Firstly, it marginalises men, who, in many ways, have a part to play in the lives of the majority of black women. Secondly, it confuses the issue of external structural economic inequality with an analysis of internal cultural traits. The effect of both these oversights has been, ultimately, to turn our attention away from looking at the importance of racial and sexual discrimination, in favour of focusing on cultural determinants to economic success or failure, and in particular has been responsible for reifying black motherhood.

This book, in which I follow the experiences of a group of young black British women as they leave school to enter the world of work, is an attempt to move away from the established emphasis on subcultural identity, towards a more structural understanding of the process of inequality. Such an account turns our attention towards the central role of the educational system in maintaining social and economic disadvantage. Chapters 3, 4 and 5, which examine the schooling experiences of young black women, focus on the institutional constraints to equality of opportunity.

To accommodate this shift towards a more structural emphasis in analysis it is necessary to re-appraise our present understanding of what is meant by educational underachievement, the black family and, in particular, black womanhood in Britain. In the context of research and writing from America and the Caribbean, a comparative consideration of the central arguments within social and educational research, race relations and feminist thought is undertaken in Chapters 2, 6, 7 and 8.

THE STUDY

This study attempted to combine a longitudinal survey approach, with what can be described as essentially a school-based ethnographic study. Despite the difficulty of combining these two distinct methodological perspectives into what may be called a 'multidimensional framework', it did offer a satisfactory means of studying the complex influences that affect the career aspirations and expectations of young black women.

The 62 young black women in this study, who were aged between 15 and 19 years, attended two comprehensive schools in south London. The girls and their black and white male and female peers, who numbered 198 in all, and who could be objectively identified as coming from working-class homes, answered questionnaires, and were interviewed and observed in their homes and classrooms over a period of 18 months.

In each school a random sample was drawn from the fifth- and the sixth-form pupils. From St Hilda's, a co-educational Catholic school, 128 (65 per cent) black and white male and female pupils were taken, whereas 70 (35 per cent) were taken from St Theresa's, a single-sex, Church of England school. Of these 62 (31 per cent) were African Caribbean young women; 13 (7 per cent) were African Caribbean young men; 77 (39 per cent) were 'other' young women; and 46 (23 per cent) were 'other' young men.

This sample, it must be stressed, was an 'observed' sample (that is, specific in its location) and therefore is not necessarily representative of the 'accessible' target population. Inferences drawn from these data therefore relate only to the population at hand and are not meant to lead to generalisations about the population as a whole.

In terms of their age, ability ranges, gender and ethnic groupings, this subpopulation of the fifth and sixth years did, however, reflect the various characteristics of the general school populations. Thus the sample had not only large numbers of girls (one school was an all-female school), but also few black males (St Hilda's, the co-educational school, was situated in an area of lower ethnic concentration).

The sample included a wide range of ethnic and racial groups not of African Caribbean origin. Because the place of birth of 94 per cent of the sample was the UK (99 per cent of black girls were British born), the ethnic origin of pupils was gauged by looking at the mothers' place of birth. Using this method 38 per cent of the sample were second-generation West Indian, 25 per cent were of Irish descent and only 27 per cent were of British parentage.

It is recognised that ethnic differences are substantial and distinctions between groups are important to make. Other second-generation, non-white pupils, though small in number, were therefore broadly classified as Asian, African, Southern European and Far Eastern. Of these 2 per cent were of Asian origin (from India and Pakistan); 3 per cent African (Nigeria and Sierra Leone), 4 per cent Southern European (Italy, Spain, Greece); and 1 per cent Far Eastern (Hong Kong and Vietnam).

Establishing the social class background of the sample was complex. The conventional procedure is to take the social class of the male head of household as representative of the social class of the family. However, for my purposes this was not an acceptable precedent as it offered no accurate way of measuring the social class of many West Indian families which were often headed by a female, even when a male was present.

It could be argued that because West Indian women so often fulfil the criteria established by conventional stratification analysts, being consistent and sustained contributors to the family income, they qualify as being eligible to define the social-class status of their families.

It was assumed, therefore, in this study that either the mother or the father, whoever could most appropriately fulfil this criterion, should define the social class of the family according to the classification system used by the Registrar General (OPCS 1980). If both the male and the female contributions were assessed as 'equal' by this criterion (that is, both worked full-time; travelled to work and so on), then the earner with the higher social class was taken to be the indicator of the family's social class, be they male or female.

Rather than introducing bias into the study, this method offers a more accurate reflection of the social and economic experience of the West Indian family. What appeared to be a completely working-class West Indian cohort if measured in terms of paternal social class, is by a culturally valid redefinition, now no longer 'objectively' classified as such. With many mothers located in social class 1 and 2 occupations these West Indian families are upwardly placed in the occupational hierarchy. It should be noted that within a redefinition of social class the family background of the white male and female pupils remains almost unchanged.

However, the working and living conditions of West Indian women in these professional occupations do not imply that they enjoy the same standards of living as whites, and in particular as white men, who are classified in similar occupational groupings (that is, qualified and well-educated nurses are in social class 2 yet paid very poorly). However, by other social-class criteria the West Indians did show differences from their white working-class counterparts; for example, they tended towards home ownership.

Using this method, 44 per cent of the black females in this study were from homes where the head of household held a professional, intermediate or managerial position; 48 per cent came from skilled manual and semi-skilled/unskilled backgrounds. Figures more accurately reflecting the dichotomy of job levels known to exist for black women in the British economy since the 1950s to the present day (*Employment Gazette* 1991).

In contrast, only 13 per cent of their female white counterparts came from professional households. The majority, 64 per cent, came from a working-class, skilled manual or semi-skilled/unskilled family background.

The sample also reflected the various ability ranges that were present in the schools. Applying the categories of the official ILEA banding system the African Caribbean pupils were, as other studies also show, disproportionately represented in the lower streams.

Among the black females 23 per cent were to be found in the high stream while 53 per cent were classified to be of low ability. No young black men were in the top stream but 77 per cent were in the lowest stream. In contrast, 44 per cent of the white female sample were high ability and 30 per cent low ability.

Other characteristics of the sample, such as family size, numbers of brothers and sisters, place of residence, male/female guardian, type of house, and experience at primary school were also investigated.

There was also a smaller random subsample of 27 younger pupils, aged 13–14 years who were in their third year of schooling. They contributed to the study by participating in informal discussions and answering 'spot' questionnaires regarding their subject and job choices.

In addition 30 young women from a school in Trinidad aged between 16 and 18 years participated in semi-structured interviews concerning their career choices and attitudes to marriage and relationships.

In youth clubs and community centres 16 young women also participated in the study. Informal discussions and exchanges with these women, aged 18+, provided additional information on the African Caribbean, British, female post-school-leaver attitudes to and experience of the labour market.

Schoolteachers, headteachers, careers officers and college staff from several institutions also contributed to the study. Interviews with them were carried out in the formal setting of their respective offices and classrooms. However, these interviews, though in formal surroundings, were not structured but focused on matters of interest.

Parents of several of the pupils also participated in the study. In-depth informal interviews were undertaken within their own homes and at meetings held in the schools.

It was a coincidence that both schools in the study had a recent history of being involved in educational research projects. As a consequence the staff in particular were familiar and at ease with the presence of a researcher and the research situation. Because of their positive relationship in the past with outside educational researchers, when approached by the ILEA, the headteachers of both schools felt uninhibited about giving me permission to carry out my research project in their respective schools.

The two schools were studied simultaneously; that is, I spent one day in one school and then the next day in the other. Depending on the time-table, some days I would spend half a day in one and the other half in the other. On other occasions I might spend several days at one school only.

General observations were made about the school, the daily regime, the headteacher's role, and so on. General staffroom observation was also undertaken, and school meetings were attended. Classroom observation constituted a major part of my time spent in the field. I attended many classes and lessons, in which my interest was not only to observe teacher–pupil interaction but other classroom situations. In particular I was interested in curriculum content and teaching effectiveness.

The observations in the school were recorded by a system of daily diary-keeping. I used short-term recall and wrote down observations, if possible at the time, but if not soon after the event, during recreation or lunch, after school, or in the privacy of the staffroom. I dated diaries and subsequently indexed them.

The questionnaire was designed primarily to obtain details of school experience and home background (including the social class of the respondent), in order to establish the factors that influence occupational aspirations and expectations of black and white, male and female pupils. It was administered to all 198 pupils in the study during their class time, and in particular their careers lessons.

The questionnaire endeavoured to place the 'objective' criteria affecting career choice, such as social and family background, culture and economic status, in the context of individual, 'subjective' preferences being made with regard to future occupations.

A postal follow-up questionnaire was sent to 72 of the young black men and women in the study four years after the initial survey. This questionnaire was designed to find out the subsequent educational and/or labour-market destinations of the pupils and was only sent to the black leavers.

Formal and semi-formal interviews were conducted at the several different sites of the study. Formal interview situations were set up in the two schools. Different groups of pupils were asked questions guided by a detailed, structured interview schedule. Each group was selected from among the pupils in the study according to their race, gender and school ability allocation. For example, some groups were all female, others just black female, while others were mixed in terms of gender and race. The interviews, undertaken with different groups of pupils, provided good 'control' conditions for interviewing. Formal interview data were taped and later transcribed.

During the year spent in the schools, informal interviews were conducted among the fifth- and sixth-year pupils contributing data of a less 'controlled' nature. Less formal interviews were also conducted elsewhere in the study. For recording informal interviews, and in an effort to maximise reliable reporting, I used both short recall and more often, note-taking, done as unobtrusively as possible if the situation allowed.

Additional data on the pupils were available in the schools from records and reports. In both schools data were also available on mock and final examinations results. Details about the pupils, such as verbal reasoning scores, punctuality, attendance, conduct and teachers' comments, were available in individual pupil records and provided an invaluable source of information.

A useful source of information on the third-year pupils came from quick, one-word, written responses to seven short questions regarding their career choices and social background. It was a simple and easy way to get structured information without administering the long, detailed and fairly complicated questionnaire. A random sample of fifth-year pupils were asked to write an essay entitled 'My Homeland'.

The case-study approach was found to be valuable in supplementing and illuminating data and observations made in other situations. Case studies of three young black women and their families were 'snowballed' from the larger sample on the basis of their willingness to co-operate.

I often visited homes, and parents were interviewed informally (sometimes other family members were interviewed if present). My method of recording informal interview data was similar to that used in the school. In the relaxed home situation where I was often regarded as a guest, it was not appropriate to use a tape recorder or to take notes, so I relied heavily on short-term recall.

Participant observation in the classroom was found to be an invaluable method of social investigation. It provided a rich source of information to complement and assist the analysis of the more quantitative longitudinal data. My position, and the sensitivity of my role as an observer in the field, meant I enjoyed a unique, yet dynamic, relationship with both the young people and the staff in the study.

 In several repects I shared much in common with my respondents. I was myself young, female, and originated from the West Indies. Having left one of the schools six years earlier, I enjoyed a unique insight into the experiences of the young black women in the study. The length of time spent in the schools (one year) and my own position as a teacher made for the formation of good relationships between myself and the staff in both schools. This position was reflected in the unconditional access I was given in both schools to records and reports.

Any subjective bias arising from my familiarity with the school, the staff, and my experiences while a pupil there must to some degree be recognised. However, it was felt that the introduction of bias this situation might encourage was far outweighed by the positive aspects of access and confidentiality that I enjoyed.

It may be assumed that the researcher's close identification with the cohort could lead to complications not only of 'internal validity', but also concerning the collection of data from other sources within the school, especially from the staff, who could have perceived the researcher as a threat. On the other hand, it can be argued that there is no way to avoid bias in the interpretation of ethnographic data. The researcher, of course, brings her own particular view of the world and the way she perceives it into the study (Mac an Ghaill 1988; Bhavnani 1991).

Stanley and Wise (1983) argue that subjectivity in feminist research is a necessary and productive input in to the study of women. The validity of personal experience, they suggest, has been submerged by the quest for 'objectivity', and as Rich (1976) argues, merely represents the term that men have applied to their subjectivity.

At a practical level, Adelman (1985) puts forward the following solution to overcome the misrepresentation so often evident in ethnographic studies. He suggests that the participant observer should be a competent member of the culture he or she is writing about. Riessman (1987) discusses the importance of shared culture and social class when interviewing women. Furthermore, it has been acknowledged that the quality of research into issues of race can greatly be improved by the interpretation and perspective brought by black scholars (Lawrence 1981; Lashley 1986).

Chapter 2

The myth of underachievement

Black girls do relatively well at school. But although the scholastic attainment of young black women has been documented it has rarely been discussed. Research investigating the educational experience of young black *people* persistently fails to integrate satisfactorily into its findings the differential achievement of black girls. In this chapter, I argue that the failure to recognise appropriately this differential educational performance has implications for research on issues of race and education.

In keeping with other research (ILEA 1987), the young black women in this study were found to do better in their final examinations than their male peers: 5 per cent received good grades in five or more subjects compared to the boys both black and white, none of whom attained such a result. Black boys did least well, 20 per cent receiving no graded result. Only 2 per cent of the black girls left school without any qualification; 93 per cent of the black girls had an average performance of between one to four passes compared to 80 per cent of the black boys and 87 per cent of the white girls and boys.

With evidence such as this, why has the phenomenon of black female scholastic success been consistently neglected for more than three decades? To answer this question it is a revealing exercise to chart the historical development of the debate on race and educational achievement. From such an exercise it becomes clear that the marginalisation of the gender issue is a consequence of the political undercurrents that have shaped research on race and education.

LAYING THE GROUNDWORK FOR NEGLECT: 1958-1970

The current neglect of black girls in educational research had its foundation over thirty years ago, in 1958. The racial unrest of 1958 was a significant watershed, not only in terms of its generally recognised political implications, but also for an influential but much less widely acknowledged reason. These race riots set in motion the wheels of what Hall (1978) describes as the 'new and indigenous racism of the post-war period'. The nature of this new British racism, characterised by white fear and hostility towards the newly arrived Commonwealth immigrants, had the effect of determining the terms of reference that have since shaped the debate on race and education; the key concepts within this perspective being race and culture (Parekh 1988). This overwhelming emphasis on race and culture meant that right from the start gender was not considered to be a major area of concern. Gender, it was believed, could not lend any valuable or illuminating insights to a debate whose underlying premise was about racial differences.

From the early to mid-1960s policy initiatives in the field of race relations were directed towards the goal of assimilation (Mullard 1982). 'Commonsense' racist assumptions about the inherent inferiority of non-European languages, family structures and life-styles determined the content of the educational developments during this period.

That little or no academic research had yet been undertaken to qualify or quantify the nature of immigrant educational needs did not inhibit the DES from producing Circular 7/65 in 1965. This controversial programme aimed at 'thinning out' the Asian and West Indian presence was guided largely by uninformed opinion as to the nature of the perceived 'immigrant problem'. The DES Circular instructed local authorities to disperse the immigrant pupil population.

This dispersal policy, commonly known as 'bussing', was racist both in philosophy and in consequence. The Circular reinforced the general and pervasive view that all Asians and West Indians, regardless of class and sex, and solely by virtue of their race, presented a problem for the education system. Thus began the exclusive focus on the black child as responsible for his (and not her) educational failure. What mattered was not whether they were male or female, but that they were black and not white.

Thus, even before any informed academic research had been undertaken, race and culture were already firmly established as the terms of reference, and as such responsible for shaping the debate on educational research for the ensuing three decades. Gender became submerged in the highly charged political exchanges that characterised this early period.

In the late 1960s, with the inception of multi-cultural education (later to be called multi-racial education), the fine tuning of racial and cultural explanations for underachievement commenced. From 1966 onwards there was a further escalation of anti-immigrant hostility exacerbated by Enoch Powell's speeches on race in 1967 and 1968. In this overall climate of hostility towards black migrants educational testing was called upon to measure scientifically the relative educational inferiority of the black child. During these early days, crude and simplistic notions of genetic intellectual inferiority were fuelled by Jensen in Britain and Eysenck in America.

This early tradition in academic research, emphasising IQ and intellectual ability by race, has been an influential undercurrent in the debate on race and education despite being publicly discredited as repugnant and insulting. Measuring differences *between* groups was clearly the order of the day in academic research on race, and not, it would seem, measuring differences *within* groups.

In 1966 research by Houghton showed for the first time that Jamaican girls were performing slightly better than boys on reasoning tests. Houghton, like other studies which followed (for example, Little *et al.* 1968; Payne 1969) showed that gender differences did exist but never explored this finding as having any significance in itself. These studies were concerned with measuring the comparative ability and performance of minority-group children and indigenous children, and little else. Females inevitably found their way into the samples by virtue of their existence in the population. However, the failure to incorporate the gender issue into these analyses cannot be regarded as a calculated omission. It is, rather, the outcome of the intellectual poverty and assumptions inherent in IQ studies. The most recent research in Britain to address the issue of IQ is a study by Mascie-Taylor and Mackintosh (DES 1985). Written over 20 years after the Houghton study, it still ignores the issue of gender differences in educational attainment.

In my discussion so far, I am not suggesting that intelligence testing can be made acceptable if black girls are included in the research. Lomax (1980) illustrates the shortcomings of research that attempts to combine the IQ perspective, albeit inadvertently, with an analysis of black females. In her study she states that while black girls were strongly motivated and had positive conceptions of themselves, they were nevertheless quite definitely intellectually more disadvantaged than other young girls.

A DECADE OF CONSOLIDATION AND THE INVISIBILITY OF GENDER: 1970-1980

Gender differences in attainment among West Indians, previously recorded in the 1960s and now known to exist, were swept aside during this era in the political undercurrents that determined the nature of the debate on race and education.

Research in the 1970s continued to refine the idea, already established in the 1960s, that poor home background, particularly adverse socio-economic circumstances, contributed greatly to low achievement among West Indian children. Only now the emphasis moved away from racial inferiority and towards social and cultural inadequacy. This was nowhere more evident than in government research and policy which reflected this national trend.

In response to the increasing inner-city unrest during the late 1960s and early 1970s, the Labour government launched a number of projects aimed at tackling the problem of urban deprivation. Both the Urban Aid Programme and the Educational Priority Projects (Halsey 1972) marked a new era in the discussion of race and underachievement. Influenced by the findings of the Plowden Report (1967) which highlighted social class deprivation, the government's Community Education Programmes of the early 1970s were not directed at alleviating racial inequality, but focused on the disadvantaged in general. Class now became the central issue on the research agenda, not race, and least of all gender.[1]

In America the 1966 Coleman Report (Coleman et al. 1969) was influential in bringing about this apparent shift towards social and cultural inadequacy as an explanation for the underachievement of the black child. Furthermore it gave impetus to the notion of negative self-esteem and negative ethnic identity that has since dominated the educational research on the black child, a notion that further established the invisibility of gender.

The idea that black children were failing for psychological reasons relative not only to middle-class but also to working-class children became a popular myth in the 1970s. It was a widely held belief that black children did not merely share the disadvantage of the indigenous working-class children but also suffered discrimination, prejudice and rejection by the dominant group (Coard 1971; Little 1975; Milner 1975, 1983). The 'commonsense' argument of what came to be known as the self-fulfilling prophecy was that black children internalise the negative racial values society has of them and as a result, regardless of whether they are male or female, come to see themselves as failures and non-achievers in schools.

Thus, by 1970 the terms of reference established in the late 1950s, race and culture, were still dominant in the debate on underachievement; only now the emphasis was less on race and inherent genetic ability, and more on culture and its presumed negative effects. An aspect of the race and education debate that contributed to the general tendency in the 1970s to overlook gender was the 'fashion' to compare West Indians' academic performance with that of their Asian counterparts. The debate was led astray by two false assumptions; namely, that *all* West Indian children fail and Asian children succeed. This 'divide and rule' philosophy suggested that there is a hierarchy of 'superior' and 'inferior' cultures. The relative cultural deprivation between ethnic groups, especially Asians and West Indians, became popular research themes and played an important role in influencing multi-cultural policy initiatives in schools.

The self-concept theorists were influential in the shaping of the multi-cultural education debate. As a consequence of their input, MCE (multi-cultural education) policy and practice took on a 're-medial' emphasis. The prescribed curriculum changes that provided the mainstay of policy initiatives were aimed at enhancing self-esteem, identified to be the source of 'the education problem'. For example, a 'special educational' concession to enhance the self-esteem of black girls was to have, in addition to their home economics curriculum, 'Caribbean flavour cooking' and 'hair braiding' (Stone 1985).

What is fundamentally inaccurate about the self-concept theory is its assumptions about the underachievement of all West Indian pupils. If black female academic success was taken into account, the basic assumption of negative self-esteem upon which the notion rests becomes questionable. It would appear, therefore, that the omission of gender renders this influential period of research focusing on negative self-esteem unreliable.

Young black women were rendered invisible in both theory and policy during this era. Black identity as the self-concept theorists described it was clearly black *male* identity. Carby (1982a) explains that in reality generalisations cannot be made about the black experience. Young black women are subject to a very different type of stereotypical image than black men. The specific image of them as unfeminine and sexually overt has consequences for the way in which black females are treated by others and the opportunities available to them.

Just as the previous decade was not completely devoid of educational research acknowledging the presence of black females, so several studies in the late 1970s commented on the differential achievement of black girls (Allen and Smith 1975; McEwan *et al.* 1975; Yule *et al.* 1975; Jones 1977; Phillips 1979; Bagley and Verma 1980; Rosen and Burgess 1980). These studies began to emerge in 1975, after a period of almost six years during which there was a complete absence of gender from educational research; six years that were, in effect, dominated by the work of the self-concept theorists.

However, none of the studies can be said to be particularly significant; for while they did acknowledge gender differences they failed to use their findings to explore new and enlightened directions in the race and education debate. The reason for this, it seems, is that none of these studies set out to address specifically the issue of black female academic achievement. Their references to gender were purely observations of a general kind about variations in their data.

YOUNG BLACK WOMEN IN EDUCATIONAL RESEARCH: A REAPPRAISAL OF CURRENT TRENDS

The acknowledgement of differential academic achievement among black girls in the 1980s and into the 1990s represents a move out of the 'dark ages' of the previous era. However, this new agenda, far from being enlightened, represents a new theoretical 'ghetto'. When studies that actually considered the issue of black females in schools began to emerge they were characterised by a distinct underlying ideological premise. This premise was the central role of the black mother. Unlike those early, distinctly pathological explanations of black disadvantage that suggested that the matriarchal structure of the black family caused it to be weak and disorganised (Moynihan 1965 in Rainwater and Yancey 1967; Gibson 1986), black achievement was now being seen as the outcome of the strong and central position of the female in the black family (Fuller 1982; Phizacklea 1982; Dex 1983; Sharpe 1987).

Both theoretical positions, though they appeared outwardly to be constructed in opposition to each other, in effect draw on two similar assumptions: the presumed matriarchal structure of the black family and the marginalisation of the black male within that structure. While the former position regarded the centrality of the females' role as 'seriously retarding the progress of the group as a whole' (Moynihan 1965 in Rainwater and Yancey 1967:76), the latter celebratory approach draws on the commonsense myth of the black females' 'tradition of self-reliance' (Phizacklea 1982).

The trend to pathologise the black female in educational research in Britain was influenced by the 1965 Moynihan Report from America (Rainwater and Yancey 1967). At the core of Moynihan's thesis on black disadvantage was the alienated and rejected black male and the mother-centred black family.[2]

In these clearly ethnocentric accounts that victimised the black woman, structural black male unemployment in America was overlooked (Ryan 1967, 1971; Davis 1982; Staples 1985). By failing to acknowledge the true significance of racial discrimination in the American labour market, education took on a special meaning in the Moynihan analysis. Education for Moynihan was the mechanism through which matriarchy was perpetuated.

Even though Moynihan is prepared to recognise openly and document the obvious academic success of black women, it is clear why he is prepared to do this. For Moynihan, black academic success is regarded as a negative rather than a positive phenomenon.

Black female achievement, which so often contradicts and upsets the established tradition of overall black underachievement, does not, in this case, detract from the argument. On the contrary, the recognition of black female academic success appears to support Moynihan's thesis. The presence of a dominant female is seen to undermine the social fabric. Thus in this context the recognition of black female academic achievement is far from enlightened.

It is unfortunate that in one of the few instances where black women are highlighted as a central force, their success should be manipulated to undermine the position of the black male. The recognition of the importance of black female academic success became sacrificed to the wider political debate on the status of the black American family. As an outcome of the Report, the Compensatory Education Programs established in America, such as Headstart, ignored black female achievement and aimed at redressing black underachievement. In America, as in Britain, policy makers failed to see black female academic success as offering a new direction in the understanding of black educational issues.

Like Moynihan, the 'progressive' cultural theorists of the 1980s emphasise matriarchy as the key to understanding black female academic success. However, unlike the cultural pathologists, they interpret this success as a positive outcome of a female-centred society. Whatever the emphasis, the fact remains that the family, and not society, is seen as the dynamic for change in both perspectives.

The strong black female as an explanatory model for the high educational aspirations of young black women, though on the surface appears 'progressive' is, however, at present both an ill-conceived and underdeveloped perspective. It represents an unsuccessful attempt to include the necessary and celebratory tradition of black women's writing[3] into educational and labour-market analysis.

An analysis that on the one hand talks about black women's 'subordinate position in economic, politico-legal and ideological relations' (Phizacklea 1982:115), but on the other hand suggests they were resisting filling such a position by 'drawing on their West Indian roots' (Dex 1983:69) does appear contradictory.

To suggest that black women possess internal and natural strengths that account for their endurance and ability to overcome the structural racism and sexism they face in the work place and in the home is naïve. Bryan, Dadzie and Scafe (1985) explain the shortcomings of these 'well-intentioned' attempts at analysing black women:

> They have tended, however, to portray black women in a somewhat romantic light, emphasising our innate capacity to cope with brutality and deprivation, and perpetuating the myth that we are somehow better equipped than others for suffering. While the patient, long-suffering victim of triple oppression may have some heroic appeal, she does not convey our collective experience.
>
> (Bryan, Dadzie and Scafe 1985: 1–2)

The 'superwoman' image of the black woman (Wallace 1978) that the 'tradition of self-reliance' presents reifies the black female experience, suggesting that she is somehow exceptional. Such a perspective implies that the dynamic which structures the black female experience is unlike that experienced by other groups in the labour market, be they black men, white women or men. While black women do have traditions of work and marriage that play an important part in understanding their working lives, this should not be confused with what is essentially a situation determined by the dynamics of an economy with a sexually differentiated labour force, fundamentally distorted by racism.

Research perspectives that stress the centrality of the matriarchal or matrifocal black family characterise many contemporary educational studies in Britain. However subtle, the pathological tradition so well-established in British research (see Carby 1982a; Lawrence 1982a, 1982b; Phoenix 1987) remains a feature of the many 'progressive' studies on black girls that have been undertaken in the 1980s: studies such as those undertaken by Driver (1980b), Fuller (1982) and Eggleston (1986).

DRIVER, RUTTER AND THE LIBERAL TRADITION

The publication in 1980 of a highly controversial report written by Geoffrey Driver entitled *Beyond Underachievement* was significant.[4] To explain the apparent academic success of West Indian girls (and the relative failure of white girls), Driver examined the respective position of women in the West Indian and British social structure. From a brief consideration of the differences he contends that in the West Indies women have a higher social and economic status than men and as such are generally regarded as the 'guardians of their family's good name' and the providers of its stable income.

His thesis appears deceptively simple. The success of black girls in British schools is attributed to the matriarchal structure of the West Indian family and their cultural life, which has been maintained by West Indians who have settled in Britain. He argues that in (white) British culture with its patriarchal structure, women have a lower status than men and are socialised to occupy subordinate social and economic roles. In West Indian culture, Driver claims that the opposite is true. It is the girls rather than the boys who are socialised to occupy superordinate positions and who are inculcated with values and expectations generally held to be conducive to educational success. In the same way that academic achievement is explained by cultural factors, underachievement is simply explained away in terms of the social structure of the the West Indian family, in a manner similar to Moynihan.

In the wake of Driver and his conclusions came another important milestone in the analysis of 'race' and underachievement. In 1982 Rutter and his team in their much publicised DES report (*Times Educational Supplement*, 8 October 1980) found that black pupils, and in particular black girls, were more likely to stay on at school after the fifth year in order to gain qualifications equivalent to those of their white peers.

The main reason for this, they suggest, was the greater commitment to education that they witnessed among West Indians. Rutter *et al.* argued that the parents' positive involvement in the education of their children was what helped the West Indian pupils to overcome the social deprivation and the negative schooling that they were more likely to experience.

Unlike Driver, Rutter *et al.* do not offer any explanation as to why black girls should be more persistent in gaining their educational qualifications compared to any of their peers. For Rutter and his colleagues the gender issue does not appear to merit any separate attention. The girls' persistence is seen only as an extension of the general West Indian commitment to education.

His emphasis on individual initiative and school-based factors overlooks the fact that schools do not operate in isolation from the rest of society. It is hardly surprising therefore to find that Rutter and his team, with their school-based explanations, are unable to do any more than acknowledge that gender differences do exist.

These two studies had little in common, although they both highlighted the presence of black achievement in schools. What they did have in common was the media interest that greeted the publication of their respective findings. The political implications of West Indian achievement were clear. That blacks were doing well was not only controversial but was also regarded as highly 'suspect' by the differing political camps, both radical and conservative. This period in educational history was marked by a mixture of hostility and indifference towards the academic performance of young black women.

BLACK FEMALE ACHIEVEMENT: THE OFFICIAL RESPONSE

The 'official' government and local authority responses to gender and race in the 1980s were characterised by both insincerity and neglect. 'Lip-service' was paid to the issue of differential achievement among black male and female pupils but nothing more was done; no 'official' research was commissioned nor was existing evidence of black female achievement integrated into policy documents and reports.

It was hardly surprising that official government reports which

n defining the problem for West Indians in Britain as
evement' should have continued to identify it as a male
These reports, it must be remembered, were written in the
wake of the black action in Brixton, Toxteth and Bristol in the early
1980s in which both the media and sociologists, black and white
alike, were reponsible for establishing the marginalisation of black
women. In the explanations for black 'disaffection' and 'alienation',
the image of youth that was presented was invariably black and male
(Cashmore and Troyna 1982; Gilroy 1981,1982; Sivanandan 1982;
Benyon and Solomos 1987).

The 1981 Rampton Report, *West Indian Children in our Schools*,
made no secret of the fact that gender was of little significance to
their investigation. The Rampton Committee, in its decision to
focus on the effects of both intentional and unintentional teacher
racism, dismissed Driver's conclusions as unsound, and in so doing
rejected the possibility of West Indian achievement. The message of
the Rampton Report was clear; underachievement, not minority
scholastic success, was the issue to be explored. With Rampton's
emphasis on negative self-esteem and the notion of the self-fulfilling
prophecy, teacher stereotypes and the operation of institutional
racism, the recognition of gender would have clearly upset their
well-defined paradigms.

Taking up the recommendations of the Rampton Report, not so
much in word as in deed, the ILEA policy statements made in 1983
emphasised the eradication of teacher racism. However, the ILEA's
definition of racism precluded the satisfactory incorporation of black
girls into their policy initiatives. In a political rather than an academic consideration, the ILEA suggested that racism and sexism are
separate but parallel experiences.

In their account of sexism in the classroom the black female
experience is overlooked as it is in their male-centred analysis of
racism in society. For the ILEA gender was distinctly a white issue
and race clearly a male matter. Because black females transcend all
three areas of 'concern' – black, working-class and female – they
become invisible by failing to comply with the rigid race, class and
sex categorisation set up by the ILEA team. As Troyna and Williams
(1986:35) suggest, this reactive approach to multi-racial initiatives
was not inspired so much by 'pedagogical foresight' as impelled
rather by more immediate political and social considerations.

The 1985 Swann Report entitled *Education for All*, like its prede-
cessor, the Rampton Report, investigated the problem of West

Indian underachievement in British schools. Its authors make clear, right from the start, that an association between gender and achievement is not a link that they wished to pursue. The authors of the Swann Report ignore the subject in their study. In the entire 806 pages of the report only 18 pages make any direct reference to girls, let alone to the wider gender issue (Mirza 1986a).

In the report Green recognises that gender has a role to play, albeit in the limited context of self-concept analysis. The DES School Leavers' Survey presents one table with a breakdown by gender. Verma's three-page summary of a longitudinal study he carried out on the effects of ethnicity on educational achievement concludes without further explanation, that 'the influence of the mother in West Indian families was particularly strong and this seemed to provide a dynamic model for the girls'. Later, in the full-length report of this study, the operation of what he calls the 'maternal interest' is never fully explained (Verma 1986).

By suggesting that there may be a gender variation in academic performance, while simultaneously casting it aside, both Rampton and Swann are indeed guilty of fulfilling the cliché that sociologists so often use, that theory, methods and ethnographic material 'neglected', 'could not find', 'cannot incorporate' or simply 'forgot' the gender element (Allen 1982).

FROM SUBCULTURES TO SUBORDINATION: BLACK GIRLS AND THE ANALYSIS OF MARY FULLER

Mary Fuller's study of black girls in a London comprehensive school is one of the few attempts to analyse the bearing which a pupil's sex and race might have on academic aspirations and achievements (Fuller 1978, 1980, 1982). Fuller confirms in her study, like those before her, the finding that differential academic outcomes exist between black boys and girls.[5] In explaining why it should be that black girls were orientated toward academic achievement, Fuller looked at the experiences of a small group of black girls in their final year of compulsory schooling.

To account for these differences, she argues that these girls formed a discernible subculture within the school. Within the context of the school the black female subculture had peculiar characteristics. She claims that it was neither one of resistance nor of conformity to the school (see also Wright 1987).

In terms of classroom behaviour, this meant that the black girls gave all the appearances of being disaffected, stating that they saw the school as 'trivial', 'boring' and 'childish'. Yet the girls, when interviewed or observed away from the classroom, were seen to be strongly committed to some aspects of schooling.

The situation as Fuller sees it is that although the girls knew their self-worth they believed this was often denied by parents and their male peers, and because of this denial, the pursuit of educational qualifications takes on special meaning. The girls did not need qualifications to prove their own worth to themselves, but rather as a public statement of something which they already knew about themselves but which they were certain was not given sufficient recognition.

Fuller argues that the forms of action by the black girls in the school were strategies for trying to effect some control over their present and future lives by proving their own worth through their academic success. Thus the structure of the subculture, she argues, emerged from the girls' positive acceptance of the fact of being both black and female. She ascertains that its 'particular flavour' was the outcome of the girls' critical rejection of the negative connotations which the categorisations female and black commonly attract.

Although Fuller's study is both a clear and stimulating account of black girls in schools, it is necessary to take issue with some of the fundamental assumptions she makes with regard to the structure and function of the subculture, and in particular her description of the influence of the black family, male peers and the role of what she calls 'double subordination' for the black girls concerned.

Fuller suggests that a major influence on the girls' feelings of isolation and anger, which in turn determine the characteristics of the subculture, is the low value of domestic work in the home and the girls' negative relationships with black male peers. However, Riley (1985) found that African Caribbean girls looked forward to relationships with men, and reported that the girls in her study felt that parents encouraged boys and girls equally. It was a sense of responsibility, and not the need to establish their self-worth, that Riley suggests gave black girls their stronger commitment to education.

Fuller, in emphasising the oppressive nature of the black family, supports the belief that cultural obstructions to fuller participation in society are reproduced within black families by black people themselves (see Foner 1979; Pryce 1979; Gibson 1986). Such assumptions are clearly the outcome of 'commonsense' pathological ideas about the black family and inappropriate definitions of sexism which have been imposed on the black experience.

The notion of 'subculture' employed by Fuller implies the central importance of 'cultures of resistance' (Willis 1977). In Fuller's work, as in so many other studies of black girls (Griffin 1985; Riley 1985; Mac an Ghaill 1988; Wulff 1988; Coultas 1989; Reid 1989), the notion of subculture has been employed because it appears to offer some understanding of creativity, activity and resistance. For example, Wulff (1988), in using the subcultural model, suggests that black girls' active pursuit of 'excitement' on the street, in clubs and in school characterised their micro-culture and structured their experience of 'growing up'.

Fuller's emphasis on 'cultures of resistance' is a problematic aspect of her thesis. Hall and Jefferson (1976) argue that to emphasise the subcultural features of youth is to divert attention away from the issues which they see as determining the quality of the experience of those being studied; issues such as unemployment, compulsory mis-education, low pay and dead-end jobs.

Fuller's use of the concept of 'cultures of resistance' results in an unrealistic, 'romantic' reappraisal of black girls' actions and decisions. Fuller's belief that these girls were highly politicised about unemployment, racism and sexism during their educational career, and planned their actions as a defiant gesture to the world, does not stand up to closer scrutiny. Research by Ullah (1985) indicated that young black women, at the point of entry into the job market, were the least aware of the groups in the study of the racism they would encounter in the work place.

In relation to black females it is necessary to incorporate not just an understanding of the girls' 'lived-out experiences' of racism in the classroom, but also an analysis of how the ideology of racism structures opportunity and limits economic horizons. It is not sufficient to demonstrate how the ideology of racism and sexism is constructed in the consciousness of individuals or groups but it must be shown how the ideology of sexually structured racism, as a dynamic and politically constructed ideology, maintains disadvantage by its effect on economic assumptions and values. Thus it is important to investigate the mechanisms of racial discrimination beyond a mere discussion of the dominant ideology and the subsequent creation of 'cultures of resistance', and to include an explanation of its operation through the various agencies, such as the school, the careers service, youth schemes and other institutions.

In addition to her subcultural analysis, Fuller employs the concept of 'double subordination' to describe what she calls the 'unique' social and economic position of black women in the economy. In Fuller's model of 'double subordination', like that of 'triple' or even 'four-fold subordination' (Morokvasic 1983), a historically specific definition of racial oppression is simply superimposed on to a culturally specific notion of sexual inequality.

This model, which has its roots in the dual systems or multi-dimensional approach to social stratification, sees gender, age, race and class as independent dimensions which cut across one another, giving rise to a complex structure of inequality (Crompton and Mann 1986). In this essentially additive and hierarchical model, inappropriately defined concepts of race, class and sex are often meaninglessly described as either 'intersecting', 'interpenetrating', 'simultaneous' or 'carried out in harness'.[6] The vague and problematic concept of 'double or triple subordination' (sometimes referred to as 'double or triple jeopardy' (King 1988) or 'whammy') appears to stem from a simple theoretical confusion. What are essentially *ideological* manifestations of oppression are described interchangeably with an *economic* evaluation of labour-market inequality. Those most ideologically oppressed may not always be the most economically disadvantaged. For example, the black female labour-market position may not always be as objectively 'disadvantaged' as the black male location (see Chapter 5).

The concept of 'double and triple subordination' presents other problems in analyses. Societies are not built up of independent dimensions or levels which are universally experienced. Carby (1982b) directs our attention to the fact that existing assumptions made by white feminists, in particular their notions of what constitutes patriarchy, the family, dependency and reproduction, become problematic when applied to the lives of black women. Bhachu (1986) also makes an important point with regard to the ethnocentricity inherent in the concepts of 'double and triple subordination'. She argues that by focusing too much on what seem to be static and unchanging traditions, the thesis of 'double and triple subordination' fails to recognise the strengths of cultural forms that can be liberating to black women. Though black women writers have been critical of the less than satisfactory theoretical treatment of black women in academic research, the matter still remains unresolved.[7]

In conclusion, Fuller's attempt to explain the academic performance of young black women, despite its theoretical shortcomings, was both pioneering in its efforts and thorough in its analysis. It marks a watershed in educational research, indicating the richness and value of a gender-orientated perspective to the study of black academic performance. It has been over a decade since Fuller first published her findings, yet in these years little *innovative* research has been undertaken to explore further the value of differential gender achievement among West Indian pupils or to investigate the racial dimension of female studies. Much of the work on black girls still remains largely influenced by the concept of subculture first employed by Fuller. Thus, while academic achievement for girls is explained in terms of subcultural resistance, for boys educational performance is still regarded as the outcome of self-concept and the self-fulfilling prophecy (Wright 1987).

FROM MATRIARCHY TO MOTHERHOOD: BLACK GIRLS IN THE EGGLESTON REPORT

The concept of the strong role model of the West Indian mother appears to have become an established part of 'commonsense' mythology concerning the black female. Hirsch (1989) warns of the dangers of idealising and mystifying a certain biological female experience and, in so doing, of reviving an identification between femininity and maternity that in the past has not served the interests of women. Though Fuller herself refers to this image of black women, the use of the strong black female role model in the Eggleston Report (1986) illustrates more aptly how this misrepresentation of black girls, originally instigated by Moynihan, has become integrated into everyday sociological thinking.

The Eggleston Report, entitled *Education for Some*,[8] is an investigation into the vocational and educational experiences of young people from various ethnic minority groups. In their conclusion, in which Eggleston and his colleagues assert that social processes in schools and society work against the efforts of young black people in Britain, the authors acknowledge that there is also a situation of differential achievement among black boys and girls.

The performance of black females in their final examinations was acknowledged to be far higher than that of black males, and equal to, if not as good as, that of white males. Because the authors do not confront the issue of gender in the Report, they in fact present confused and contradictory statements as to why this difference should occur. The Report claims that obstacles to equitable entry to examinations are an important factor in explaining the maintenance of black underachievement. To have asked the question why African Caribbean girls should be more likely to be entered for specific examination subjects than boys, or to have investigated the way in which the black male experience of racism differs from that of the girls, would surely have been appropriate in an investigation of young *people's* educational and vocational situations. By black underachievement Eggleston *et al*. must surely, by their own criteria, mean black *male* underachievement.

The aspirations of the young women studied in the Eggleston Report, unlike their academic attainment, is given some marginal consideration. In a two-page (pp. 93–4) analysis, the concept of motherhood and the strong black female role model is implied when accounting for the incidence of high occupational aspirations among the 38 African Caribbean girls in the study. They suggest that, like their mothers, black girls wish to 'better themselves'.

An unqualified assumption appears to be being made about the central influence on African Caribbean girls' occupational aspirations. The authors point to a link between the mothers' occupational status and that of their daughters' aspirations. However, in making such a connection they are acknowledging the thesis that black females exhibit a form of cultural strength and resourcefulness that they transmit to their daughters who wish to emulate the strong role model provided. This emphasis not only marginalises the male, it also fails to investigate the influence of the labour-market structures that determine the job opportunities for migrant women and their children.

A further common misrepresentation made by Eggleston *et al*. in their Report concerns the notion of West Indian girls' attitudes toward their own motherhood and careers. They suggest that because African Caribbean girls are more likely than any of their peers to take as little time off work as possible when having a child, they are more 'careerist'. By suggesting that such a response indicates that they are 'careerist' is inappropriate for several reasons.

The authors' interpretation of the girls' desire to remain at work as 'careerist' implies that they consider that there is a singular, universal orientation to work shared by all the girls irrespective of their racial and class background. It should be noted that black girls may not regard having children and continuing to work in the same way as their white peers. For many West Indian women, to work and bring up children is not so much a 'careerist' choice as a historical necessity.

In conclusion, the Eggleston Report, while occasionally referring to young women in its statistical data, does not attempt to integrate a gender analysis into the investigation of ethnic differences. Thus Eggleston *et al.* present a thesis whose claims to investigate *black youth* cannot be verified as the experiences of *black females* are overlooked.

GENDER AND THE WORK OF THE BLACK 'SELF-CONCEPT' CRITICS

In the late 1970s and early 1980s another trend emerged in educational research that made black girls more visible. The studies of two black sociologists in particular, Delroy Louden (1978, 1981) and Maureen Stone (1985 (1981)), included the experiences of black female pupils in their work. These writers, in their efforts to challenge the 'self-concept' theorists' notion of negative black self-esteem, employed evidence provided by the actions and beliefs of black girls.

However, because Louden and Stone were attempting to refute an established school of thought they had little choice but to adopt the traditional terms of reference, 'race and culture', from which to launch their own attack. This fact, more than any other, inhibited the extent to which black females could be incorporated into their studies. Thus both authors, rather than integrating gender into their analysis, used their findings on girls to demonstrate the point that high black self-esteem does exist among all black pupils, and particularly the girls. This period of research was important as it demonstrated differences between boys and girls of the same racial origin, which had so often been ignored in the work of the self-concept theorists of the 1970s.

STATISTICAL SURVEYS AND EMPIRICAL EVIDENCE

Although not specifically aimed at West Indian girls, empirical and statistically orientated research has dominated the most recent efforts to investigate the black female situation. National surveys and large-scale empirical studies provide further evidence that young black women have differential experiences in education and the labour market which contrast with those of both their male and white female peers. The ongoing Labour Force Surveys (Central Statistical Office 1991; OPCS 1985,1987; *Employment Gazette* 1985,1987, 1990,1991) and the Policy Studies Institute (PSI) studies (Brown 1984; Smith and Tomlinson 1989), for example, show the educational and occupational characteristics of young black women on a nationwide basis. Reports by the DES, the DOE and the ILEA[9] which include a breakdown of their results by gender, provide detailed studies suggesting that generalisations about the outcomes for all black pupils cannot be made.

There has been much concern within the black community about the collection and use of empirical data on racial matters, and not without cause (Burney 1988). Although the issue of ethnic monitoring is recognised as problematic, and misrepresentation in statistical fact-gathering is often common, the data that have been collected on black females are rich sources of information, revealing patterns that many of the more interpretative studies we have discussed so far have failed to acknowledge. The patterns emerging from the figures show black women of all ages to be committed to further and continuing education, to be better qualified than black males and to be more active in the labour market than their white female counterparts.

The findings of the DES School Leavers Survey 1981/82 (DES 1985:110) with regard to gender are clear. From their statistical presentation the authors conclude:

> West Indian children, more especially the girls, also tend to stay on longer than other children . . . they also tend to go more frequently than the average child from school to some form of full-time education course – but not to university or to pursue a degree course – and to have obtained a lower general level of academic achievement at school.
>
> (DES 1985:116)

Similarly, the ILEA Research and Statistics Report on examination results and ethnic background (ILEA 1987:7,19) observes that in all ethnic groups girls did better. African Caribbean girls were notably performing much better than African Caribbean boys, and even the white boys.[10]

Although Sillitoe and Meltzer (1985) employ a more interpretative account in their study of West Indian school leavers in London and Birmingham, the statistical information they provide with regard to gender is useful. Their investigation into career aspirations show the similarities and differences between West Indian males and females, indicating that, while West Indians in general were more ambitious than whites, the girls showed a marked preference for non-manual work compared to the boys' desire for skilled manual work (p. 46). Sillitoe and Meltzer also note that in conjunction with 'high ambitions', black girls showed a 'striking enthusiasm' for part-time further education, especially in contrast to white females, and taking into consideration the difficulties they encountered in getting time off from work to undertake such studies (p. 98). However, in seeking to explain their observation Sillitoe and Meltzer make many of the 'commonsense' assumptions that we saw earlier in the Eggleston Report. Links are made between mothers' work and daughters' aspirations purely on the basis of an 'educated' guess rather than considered investigation.

The third PSI Survey, *Black and White in Britain* (Brown 1984), gives a detailed and informative account of living and working conditions for black people in Britain. In so doing it is one of the few studies that gives substantial consideration to the characteristics of West Indian female experiences. With regard to education Brown declares:

> It is notable that West Indian women are involved in part time study to a greater extent than Asian and White women . . . . The spread of qualifications pursued by West Indian women is very broad: 18 per cent of them are studing for 'O' level, 25 per cent for clerical or commercial qualifications, 10 per cent for a degree, 10 per cent for City and Guilds exams and 6 per cent for nursing exams.

> (Brown 1984:136)

Evidence such as this shows not only the levels of commitment but, more importantly, the results of restricted access to educational opportunity (that is, black women have to return to get basic qualifications and few actually achieve the privilege of a university education). The PSI evidence also helps dispel many myths, such as the belief that nursing is a preferred profession among skilled and educated black women. As such it confirms the influence of the labour market in shaping the destinations of many black women in contemporary Britain.

The 1986–1988 Labour Force Survey gives a picture of overall statistical trends for black people in general but also provides a useful breakdown according to gender. It shows the extent of disadvantage encountered by West Indian men and women when compared to their white counterparts of equivalent qualifications, age and sex. The survey also reveals the reproduction of disadvantage within the second-generation males and females by examining their high and disproportionate rates of unemployment in the context of their improved levels of education.

For example, West Indian females aged 16–24 had an unemployment rate of 21 per cent. West Indian males aged 16–24 had a rate of 31 per cent, while their white male peers only experienced 16 per cent, with white females 14 per cent. The employment experience of the parents of these West Indian youths, who, as the Labour Force Survey points out were less qualified than their children, is clearly determined by different labour-market demands over time. West Indian males 45–64 years old had an unemployment rate of 18 per cent and West Indian females 45–59 years old had a rate of 10 per cent (OPCS 1987). This still compared unfavourably to their white counterparts' experiences: white females over 45 had an unemployment rate of 6 per cent, and males of 8 per cent.

The data provided by the Labour Force Survey is useful, as it puts the black female experience into a comparative context. It shows that regardless of qualifications or aspirations, black women (who often had the higher and more determined record of attaining such qualifications) like their male peers suffered substantial disadvantage and discrimination in the job market. At the same time it also shows that their experience differed in kind from their black male and white female peers.

Thus it is clear from our discussion of empirical research that, while black females struggle to do well, the constraints of the economic and political environment in which they live severely curtail whatever achievements and aspirations they might have.

CONCLUSION: A HISTORY OF NEGLECT

What has been illustrated in the review of the early literature on race and education in Britain is that the terms of reference that shaped the debate on race and education since its beginnings in the 1950s remained firmly established. These terms of reference, politically defined as 'race and culture', encouraged a perspective that resulted in gender being marginalised in the educational analysis of underachievement. Comment on black female performance was either absent from, or if noted, simply ignored in such research areas as diverse as IQ, self-concept, cultural and socio-economic disadvantage. The consequence of this oversight was more far-reaching than is often acknowledged. By failing to recognise the significance of differential achievement, research on racial and educational issues confined itself to specific avenues of investigation – avenues that often perpetuated ill-defined or unsubstantiated theoretical explanations for West Indian underachievement.

Studies of the 1980s that do take account of black females, though they vary in substance and in kind, all agree that black girls not only have high aspirations but also higher levels of academic attainment than their male peers. However, because underachievement has remained the overriding concern of educational research with regard to the black child, this observation, as indeed the whole matter of gender, has been marginalised in the academic debates.

In studies that do address the issue of black scholastic success, boys are clearly overlooked. For example, Eggleston and Driver associate high aspirations among West Indian girls with the strong role model of the mother. Fuller, on the other hand, suggests that positive orientation to education can be explained by a black female subculture of resistance. Boys, who it is assumed are not affected by their parental orientation, least of all by any maternal influence, are thus not regarded as part of the equation. Unlike the girls, who are seen as part of a privileged and select club, they remain subject to the injustices of institutional racism and victims of the self-fulfilling prophecy of failure and underachievement.

Finally, the question remains as to why the gender issue should be perceived so negatively.[11] The answer appears simple. The spectre of achievement among some blacks, or blacks up to a certain age, or in particular schooling environments, would suggest that a radical reappraisal of contemporary thinking on the subject is essential. Rather than focusing on the family, parental social status, economic and social disadvantage, IQ, poor self-concept and ethnic self-esteem, commentators on the issue may have to address the far more controversial matter of the fundamental social inequality in British society.

Chapter 3

Do schools make a difference?

In their research Rutter *et al.* (1979) asked the question, 'Do schools make a difference?' They found that individual schools do make a difference on the basis of how they are run. Discipline, uniform, punctuality are some of the indicators they employed to measure in what way a school can achieve a better outcome. However, not all studies accept this argument. Jencks *et al.* (1972) provide evidence to the contrary. They suggest that because of the social and economic inequality that exists between pupils, schools in fact can make very little difference to educational outcomes.

This debate, academic though it may seem, is important in our investigation of young black women's educational outcomes. Young black women are highly motivated to the goal of academic credentialism, yet their educational performance does not necessarily reflect their level of academic motivation. Such a finding suggests that there could be a connection between the schooling process and educational performance.

The evidence presented in the following pages shows, from a comparative evaluation of the two schools in the study, that there were considerable differences in educational outcome between them.

In order to address the issues that the conflicting theses of Jencks and Rutter raise with respect to young black women, we must consider to what degree the differences in educational outcome between the schools are a consequence of the school itself, in terms of how it is run, or due to the variations in the social and cultural background of the pupils within its classrooms (see Drew and Gray 1991). To do this we must examine the daily running of the school, its efficiency, its use of resources, its objectives, aims and approaches to the schooling of its pupils and its orientation to the labour market.

THE SCHOOLS[1]

St Hilda's was a co-educational, Catholic school situated in the inner London Borough of Southwark. St Theresa's was a single-sex (girls only), Church of England school located in the neighbouring borough of Lambeth.[2]

They were average-sized comprehensives with approximately 700 pupils, and class sizes of about 25–30 pupils. Both schools drew their pupils from the locality and, despite their religious orientation, the intake appeared to reflect the social and ethnic make-up of the boroughs in which they were situated.

St Hilda's pupils came from the Catholic community of Southwark and in particular the Camberwell area (90 per cent of the pupils from St Hilda's came from the local area). St Theresa's had as its catchment the Brixton and Norwood areas of Lambeth (84 per cent of its pupils came from the local area), and although nominally a Church of England foundation, had a mixed intake of all religions and ethnic groups.

At St Theresa's 53 per cent of the school's population was of West Indian origin. In contrast to St Theresa's, only 18 per cent of St Hilda's population was of West Indian origin. Because of its Catholic emphasis, St Hilda's had a fair proportion of 'white minorities', such as the Irish and Southern Europeans (Italian and Spanish).

The two schools were also situated in boroughs characterised by all the social and economic indicators of inner-city decline and deprivation. In terms of poor housing, unemployment, educational deprivation and restricted labour-market opportunities for men and women, these two boroughs scored highly.

The schools themselves were examples of the contrasting standards in building stock that characterise inner-city comprehensive schools. St Hilda's was situated on a busy main road, next door to a large bus depot. The school itself was enclosed by a high fence made of wire. The school entrance, surrounded by unwelcoming metal bars and a heavy metal gate, opened on to a path flanked on either side by tarmac play areas. The lack of any grass or trees added to the school's austere and dilapidated appearance. The building itself consisted of a series of dull pink and yellow pre-fabricated extensions around a main modern building. Several of the panels that made up these buildings had been vandalised, many being 'kicked in' or painted on.

St Theresa's, in sharp contrast, was situated in pleasant 'green' surroundings. The front of the building was dominated by the façade of an old house. A dual driveway swept up to the front entrance, and carefully tended gardens and the large green playing fields gave the impression that the school was far away from the reality of its immediate location. The school, despite its environment, was situated near to several large post-war and modern council estates and within walking distance of the city centre of Brixton.

EXAMINATION RESULTS

St Hilda's final examination performance showed a markedly different pattern from that of St Theresa's. The most able pupils at St Hilda's performed less well than the most able pupils at St Theresa's. It was found that whereas 65 per cent of St Theresa's top set pupils (Band 1) gained good passes in five or more 'O' level and CSE subjects, only 19 per cent of St Hilda's most able pupils did as well.

However, the differences between the schools were far less marked when the results of the lower-ability pupils were compared, although a notable difference still remained. Of St Theresa's pupils 44 per cent classified as of average ability (Band 2) received average passes (that is, passed at least one subject but got not more than four passes of good grades), whereas only 32 per cent of St Hilda's Band 2 pupils received the same grade.

Low-ability (Band 3) pupils fared badly in both schools, again those at St Hilda's being worse off. At St Hilda's 28 per cent of the pupils left before sitting their final exams compared to 6 per cent at St Theresa's. Of those who remained 24 per cent at St Theresa's received the lowest graded CSE result, compared to 16.7 per cent of Band 3 pupils at St Hilda's.

What seemingly characterised the results of St Theresa's was a form of 'academic selectivity'. This apparent selectivity was the outcome of the obvious nurturing of those pupils in Band 1 at the expense of the average pupils in Band 2, and especially of those least able in Band 3. This was illustrated by the fact that the performance scores of the Band 1 pupils were 28.8 points higher than those in Band 3.

St Hilda's displayed a different type of regime, one that neither specifically encouraged nor cared for those of high ability or those of less ability. This form of 'academic mediocrity' did not produce academic excellence among its best pupils nor even everyday enthusiasm among its least able students. Here the performance score was only 18.9 points higher for the Band 1 pupils than for the Band 3; a much less obvious distinction than for St Theresa's 28.8 points.

The distinctive regimes in both of the schools, which greatly affected educational outcomes for not only the black girls but all pupils, appeared to be directly related to the attitude and orientation of the individual headteacher. The evidence gathered that indicated this causal link between educational outcome and headteachers' leadership was obtained not only from the heads themselves in interviews and conversation, but also from written reports,[3] interviews with staff and staff meetings.

ST HILDA'S: A CASE OF ACADEMIC MEDIOCRITY

The HMIs noted in their 1984 Quinquennial Report that at St Hilda's: 'The underachievement of able pupils [namely, Band 1 at 11+ entry] is a major problem which all teachers should tackle' (p. 2). The report goes on to recommend that in order to rectify the situation – that is, to stretch the more able and support the less able – the headmaster, Mr Madden, together with his three deputy headteachers, should 'reconsider their overall management of St Hilda's, with regard to leadership, oversight and supervision of staff' (p. 2).

In a not dissimilar argument from that outlined by Mortimore *et al.* (ILEA 1986a), what the HMIs appear to be suggesting in their recommendations is the need for a more purposeful leadership from the head. They were supported on this issue by the staff in general, who often complained about Madden's relaxed and often ineffectual approach to his responsibilities as head of the school. The teachers' complaints focused on aspects of St Hilda's that were highlighted in more general terms in the Quinquennial Report as areas of weakness in the regime. I shall now turn to a consideration of these shortcomings within St Hilda's that accounted for its overall state of academic mediocrity.

1 Discipline and control

St Hilda's was a school that had its fair share of social problems – a reflection of its situation in a declining area of the inner city. However, many of these problems in the school were exacerbated not only by Madden's ineffectual approach to discipline, but also by his lack of awareness about everyday matters. For example, he was not in control of the violent local gang wars that spilled over into the school (there had been several fights and even a stabbing nearby). There was also tension between pupils of rival Catholic schools in the area. The alarming rate of non-attendance was another issue. In one fifth-year class at least six pupils were non-attenders. There were four pregnancies in one year, and glue sniffing was a serious problem, as was vandalism.

The head, Mr Madden, was a small, pleasant, middle-aged man with a sense of humour, as he demonstrated on our first meeting in his office:

> You are probably wondering what this is [*points to a bottle of blue liquid on his desk*]; well, it's my secret weapon. Chewing-gum remover! I look for gum on desks, walls, I find it invaluable as a head . . . I can go round with the excuse that I am looking for chewing gum . . . it's PR. It helps break down the authority image of the head. I get to know them and they me. It is important that you are not seen as some one up there.

Whatever the outcome of his unconventional approach to public relations within his school, he was considered by both pupils and staff to be a somewhat eccentric personality, as one member of staff said: 'The pupils don't like him, they think he is a bit of a fool. There is no real contact or understanding between them and him' (Mr Gavin: Mathematics teacher). His eccentricity was further illustrated by his response to the presence of a 'flasher' on the school premises who had been 'showing himself' to the girls and female members of staff. This had been going on for over a week but when it was reported to Madden and suggested that the police should be brought in he laughed, and said, 'Not to worry, I'm sure it's harmless. He probably just likes little children, that's why he comes.'

As St Hilda's was a large, inner-city comprehensive school there were a series of observable consequences that arose from his unusual attitude to discipline, control and authority. It was apparent that discipline was a real problem at St Hilda's. The Quinquennial Report had this to say with regard to the matter: 'A school policy needs to be developed . . . we noted a feeling that procedures with regard to difficult children need to be strengthened' (p. 6). Staff did indeed often complain about the lack of a referral procedure. For example, for over two years Dr Ashraf had had a troublesome fifth-year class. Three boys were particularly disruptive and unpleasant. Despite several complaints to the head no action had been taken, because among other things,[4] as Dr Ashraf explained, there was no proper system of punishment in the school:

> They should have been removed, made to sit somewhere in the public eye but there is no such facility. There should be a room with some sort of supervision. But there is no room, no teacher, no central organised system. . . . They just carry on two years making life hell [sic].

There was a great deal of evidence to suggest that the lack of discipline in the school affected not only the morale of the staff but also presented a problem to the pupils, who were constantly having their lessons disrupted by those who chose to do so. I recorded many incidents of fights or bad behaviour in the lessons (such as jumping on tables and swearing, walking about and so on). Often teachers would turn a blind eye and proceed with the class as a means of coping with a continually recurring situation. One teacher described how she felt about the lack of discipline and the unpleasant school environment it created:

> When I first came here I felt ill. I used to go home and throw up. This place was and is awful. . . . In the corridors, you notice, no pupil 'sees' you, let alone talks to you. There is no friendliness here, this really struck me when I first came. In fact I would describe it as a hostile place.
>
> (Ms Phillips: head of the English department)

2 Homework

Discipline was not the only shortcoming at St Hilda's. There were other aspects of Mr Madden's leadership that could be seen to be directly related to the mediocre educational outcomes so evident at the school, as the Quinquennial Report indicated in its discussion about schoolwork and in particular homework:

> The detailed specifications for homework for each year group should be established by the deputy head teacher for curriculum matters. Present procedures are unsatisfactory. . . . Evident slackness in this area may well be contributing to the underachievement of many pupils.
>
> (p. 3)

The lack of structured homework was apparent. During lessons very few pupils were given assignments or, if they were, they rarely completed the work, a weak excuse often being accepted as adequate. One teacher complained:

> Mr Madden said once, 'Give homework', but then, you won't believe this, he said, 'Give homework because it keeps the children off the streets and because parents like to see it and it gives a good image for the school.' Well, I always thought homework was for the benefit of education, not just a function of discipline or for the image of the school.
>
> (Ms Cole: Religious and General Studies teacher)

Ms Bell, another teacher, pointed to a consequence of this relaxed approach to homework for the pupils concerned: 'You find that they just cannot cope with homework. They even need help to fill out their homework sheets. They have no idea how to organise their learning.'

3 The curriculum

Under the Madden regime there were other educational practices that went on which, as the Inspectorate stated, were not only detrimental to the educational performance of the pupils in general, but to Band 1 in particular (where 25 per cent of the black girls were concentrated). Again they write: 'We think the abandonment of the compulsory practical subject is a retrograde step . . . low performance of Band 1 pupils may be caused by this factor (if the teaching is not carefully adapted to different examination syllabuses).'

A report by Hargreaves (1984) to the ILEA reinforces the need for a structured curriculum, the wisdom of which was clearly being ignored by Mr Madden in his alternative strategy. Despite the adoption of a less structured curriculum, the pupils both at the third-year stage of option choices and later during the crucial years of the fifth and sixth form often found themselves without the support necessary to maintain such a policy successfully. On the whole, pupils often found themselves ill-advised.

Furthermore, pupils were not encouraged to take a science subject. Madden's influence over the curriculum was significant. He refused Ms Cole, the Religious and General Studies teacher, permission to have any comparative input into her lessons, adhering to his conviction that multi-racial education was unnecessary. Moreover, recent issues in curriculum development were notably absent at St Hilda's, apparent in a lack of innovation in the teaching content and method. The many lessons that I observed were often dull and uninteresting, the outcome being bored, non-responsive or sometimes disruptive pupils.

4 Examinations

At St Hilda's there was an obvious absence of an 'exam ethos'. During the months preceding the final summer examinations the young black women in this school often complained about the lack of support and assistance. During this usually tense time of the school year, the atmosphere at St Hilda's, in the classrooms, staffrooms and school generally, seemed remarkably relaxed and 'panic-free'. Ms Ward, a recent addition to the staff of St Hilda's, had this to say about her fifth-year English class, in which there were several Band 1 black girls:

> The fifth form I just left was so advanced comparatively to this, much more serious. The whole school was 'geared up' for the exams, here no one seems to care. I wish I still had my old 'O' level class, with this lot it is a lot more boring, I can tell you. I have to do all the groundwork as they have done nothing so far. Only the poems on the syllabus and it is March already. Nothing, absolutely nothing. It is boring for them too. They have no idea, one girl said to me, 'Why do we have to do all these poems? I know the one I want to answer in the exam.' So unrealistic, they have no idea about exams, what if that one doesn't come up?

The lack of 'exam fever' apparent in the other school in the study was not only notably absent from the pupils but was also reflected in the staffroom. The staff in general were not anxious about the performance of 'their' pupils, as were their colleagues at St Theresa's. In fact, the exams were not even discussed, except in the context of their being a nuisance. Staff openly expressed their annoyance at having to come in during exam time when there was no teaching to do.

This lack of commitment towards the pupils was widespread. In the staffroom, in sharp contrast to the other school in the study, the welfare of pupils, either individually or generally, was hardly ever discussed, as were school issues or policy. There was very little professional interaction between staff, who on the whole sat day in and day out in the same mutually exclusive groups. If teachers were not pursuing their own individual tasks of marking or lesson preparation, they were to be found engaged in lighthearted exchanges about non-school events. For example, there was a group of young male teachers who always sat together and discussed only football, TV, and so on but never pupil welfare or school issues.

It was evident that teachers were also less than conscientious about their teaching tasks in other ways too: getting off early or avoiding any extra duty assigned to them (during school hours). One teacher remarked:

> Few teachers are committed here. They say, why bother? Some teachers are just bullies here and such bad teachers, they are awful to the pupils. It's a wonder they get anything out of them. Some staff go home early on a Friday and no one says anything. Madden, I doubt he even knows. Yesterday I stayed till 11.30 [p.m.] and the day before, 9.30 [p.m.]. I get a headache by Friday I'm so exhausted; I think, what's the point?
>
> (Ms Reed: Social Studies and Careers mistress)

This general malaise, it could be suggested, can be attributed to the lack of accountability of the staff to the head. Communication between Madden and his colleagues was restricted by his practice, even though he claimed otherwise, of a hierarchically structured system of authority.

5 Decision making

The unequal, but badly organised, distribution of power within the school not only affected the level of staff accountability but also their involvement in the decision-making process. The Quinquennial Report noted several times the marked lack of staff enthusiasm and involvement in matters concerning consultation and decision making. The HMIs observed: 'The Academic Committee appears to be less successful in dealing with its areas of concern. Although the meetings of the Committee are open to all staff, few teachers who are not heads of department attend' (p. 6). For that matter, staff were rarely present at any meetings that were not compulsory. As one teacher explained, Madden himself did not attend more meetings than he had to.

> Madden, he is so incompetent, he doesn't talk to anyone or discuss anything with anyone and no one with him. . . . There are

so many committees set up for us to see to. That's his job – but because he is so useless it's left up to others and in the end no one really cares.

(Mr Jarvis: Biology teacher)

6 Leadership

The effect of poor leadership by the head on the staff of St Hilda's was acknowledged in the Quinquennial Report: 'We take the view that work of the teachers could with advantage be subject to more co-ordination and supervision . . . . once decisions are taken it is essential they are adhered to by all. We noted a lack of uniformity' (p. 7). The HMIs proceed to give examples of how this lack of leadership can filter down and impinge on the quality of the teaching. Following on from the statement quoted above they write:

Perhaps some examples would make the point. We found it surprising that in a school where underachievement of able pupils is a priority, so many teachers ignore the homework time-table. One such fifth-year pupil who had attended regularly, had been set only seventeen homework sessions out of a possible fifty-nine during the first half of term. Equally disturbing, in an authority which is generous in its allocation of capitation, is that some departments are apparently short of such basic items as textbooks.

(p. 7)

This was not the only way in which the impoverished leadership provided by Mr Madden manifested itself. The lack of inter-departmental communication it produced led to an absence of efficiency brought about by the limited and often irrational pooling of financial and other resources. The Quinquennial Report suggests that this failure had much to do with the role of the head in co-ordinating change. They write:

The Resources and Academic Committees could link with the Heads of Department and Year Committee. There is in our view no substitute for a headmaster meeting regularly with his Heads of department and the pastoral Heads at properly constituted meetings to consult about major matters, to establish school policy and procedures, and to ensure full implementation.

The outcome of 'this unfortunate division between the academic and pastoral life' within the school meant that truancy and the high rate of post-16 school leavers (a major problem in the school), was considered neither the responsibility of the pastoral department nor the academic body. Inadequate record keeping also meant that effecting the school's smooth change-over to mixed-ability teaching was greatly handicapped.

Mortimore *et al.* (ILEA 1986a) suggest that inadequate leadership can bring about instability within the school. This appeared to be the case at St Hilda's. Though some teachers had been there for many years,[5] especially those with a strong Catholic affiliation, staff turn-over was high. On the whole, few teachers had been there long, and in the eighteen months that I was there not only was absenteeism high, but several members of staff also left. Some left not to be replaced.

For example, the Computing and Business Studies department had no teacher for a year after the previous member of staff had become unwell. The pupils in this class had had no tuition during that year, had worked on their own and were now being entered for the examination. The Religious Education teacher left one month before the final examination. It was two weeks before a supply teacher was sent in to replace her. There was an obvious lack of concern about the urgency of replacements by the headmaster.

The fact that the staff lacked a 'common theme', as one teacher suggested, could be put down to the lack of good leadership. Indeed, Mr Madden showed little or no interest in many contemporary issues, as the HMIs observed:

> The school does not appear to be tackling with sufficient vigour the range of problems encompassed by the Authorities' Policy Papers on multi-ethnic education . . . in several year groups children of West Indian origin were over-represented in the lower streams.
>
> (p. 3)

As already discussed earlier in this chapter, the issue of MRE was regarded as unnecessary by Mr Madden, a point which he made quite clear: 'We know what we are about here. . . . We don't need anyone telling us how to run our affairs.' Madden's lack of support for this issue filtered through to the rest of the staff who, taking their lead from him, hardly ever attended any MRE meetings. One member of staff, who later left the school, commented on the general state of affairs at St Hilda's regarding this lack of innovation as symptomatic of a broad state of apathy: 'There is no direction here, you don't feel part of a movement. My department never does anything together' (Mr Lewis: Social Studies teacher).

The headmaster only involved himself in matters that he found relevant, and it appeared that the most important aspect of the school was its religious function. Madden attended to his duties rigorously in this respect. The Quinquennial Report did remark on the positive orientation of the school in this regard: 'We would like to record that the ethos of St Hilda's is clearly one of a Christian school' (p. 2).

Madden's infrequent visits to the staffroom were nearly always concerned with church-related matters. He had a particularly close working relationship with the religiously involved members of staff, with whom he formed a definite 'clique' (for example, Sister Margarita). During my time 'in the field', the only issue that aroused Mr Madden to anger was the embarrassingly poor attendance at the Wednesday afternoon Penitence service.[6]

Summing up the evidence presented here it could be argued that 'academic mediocrity' at St Hilda's was the outcome of lack of a purposeful leadership, which in turn affected staff morale, standards of teaching and the overall school climate. This causal observation is very much in keeping with the findings of Mortimore et al. that:

> Indicators of the heads' positive leadership, especially in connection with academic matters were significantly related to teacher behaviour . . . positive school climate was closely linked to various aspects of teacher behaviour.
>
> (Mortimore et al.: ILEA 1986a)

ST THERESA'S: A CASE OF ACADEMIC SELECTIVITY

> There's a major problem at this school, that you can't help but notice. This school has never faced up to the fact that it is now comprehensive.
>
> (Mr Ellis: Advisory Teacher for 38 schools in Southwark and Lambeth)

Mr Ellis's observations were not unfounded. Evidence obtained during my time spent at St Theresa's revealed the presence of a two-tiered system of education. It was clear that the quality of education received by the girls of high ability was markedly superior to that received by those of less ability. Not only did the examination results reveal this double standard, but so did the attitude of the staff and in particular the orientation of the headmistress, Ms Grey.

1 Recruitment

In the school's Quinquennial Review (1977–1982) published and presented to the Governors in 1984, Ms Grey's underlying attitude towards the change-over from a grammar to a comprehensive system is apparent. In the following extract she expresses her reservations when describing the 'new intake':

> During the past five years the nature of the intake to the school has changed radically; our pupils now come from a much wider range of social and ethnic backgrounds than formerly and we are taking our share of disturbed and difficult pupils.
>
> (p. 5)

She goes on to elaborate on the way in which this change has affected the make-up of the school and inadvertently suggests ways to remedy the situation.

> The proportion of pupils whose families are of Afro-Caribbean origin has greatly increased and is now well over 50 per cent; as a Grammar school it was less than 10 per cent. The majority of our pupils now come from working-class families . . . some middle-class parents do not care for the present social and ethnic mix of the school.
>
> (p. 28)

Ms Grey suggests that a way to counter the falling numbers of pupils who apply to enter the school is to demonstrate to parents that, in spite of the new intake, 'the school continues to provide a good education'. It is implicit in this statement that *good* schooling means *grammar* schooling.

Many members of staff (many of whom had been there before the 1977 reorganisation) also were of the opinion that the racial and social intake was in itself a cause of problems for the education of the pupils. Ms Warr, the Religious Studies teacher, made this very clear:

> Another problem is presented by the large intake of children from West Indian Pentecostal Churches. . . . This has created a teaching problem for the department staff and a learning problem for the children concerned. At present the problem remains unresolved.
>
> (p. 129)

Statements such as these show that there was little willingness on the part of many to adapt to the changes demanded by a new and different pupil intake. This lack of flexibility, the desire to resist change and retain the characteristics of a grammar school, was a central feature of St Theresa's. Comprehensivisation was continually associated with the 'new and difficult' (mainly black) intake. Ms Grey and her staff often referred to the social and cultural problems now facing the school since its change-over:

> Most West Indians are one-parent families, the girls have a lot of cooking and working to do and that influences their school work. We have many problems now, particularly with the fifth [33 per cent black]. Groups of them are being very naughty, disruptive, and their parents are needed.
>
> (statement by Ms Grey)

The entry requirements of St Theresa's that ensured that the majority of lower-ability pupils were more likely to be recruited from ethnic minority backgrounds reinforced the staff's image that black pupils have learning difficulties.

These requirements were hierarchically stated: (1) that the girls must be Church of England. If not, they must be (2) practising Christians, or (3) have a sister already there. They would take non-Christians (that is, Muslims) and any other candidate who did not fulfil the first three requirements for their lower-ability classes.

These criteria were not often met in that order by the West Indians. As most West Indians tended to be Pentecostal, that reduced their chances considerably of being in Band 1 (most of the Band 1 pupils who tended to be Church of England were white). Because of the comparative youth of the black population in the UK many girls were the eldest sibling so they were not recruited under the third criterion.

2 The school climate

It was the 'bright' girls who benefited from the on-going grammar-school ethos that characterised the school and pervaded the staff-room. As Mr Ellis observed: 'One plus about this school is its grammar past. It has its good sides. It is self-assured about itself as a school.'

Ms Grey was a direct 'no-nonsense' sort of person. She had been at the school for well over fifteen years, the last seven as head, previously having served as deputy head. Though she had taught when St Theresa's was a grammar school, she had presided over its comprehensivisation. Many members of staff who had been there before its change-over still remained. The staffroom, which was a small and friendly place, was a hive of activity with a great deal of pre-lesson preparation going on.

Staff conversations, which were often involved, concerned among other things issues about pupils and the school. Ms Grey had a close and informed relationship with her staff and exercised a great deal of influence over them. She would find time in her busy schedule to come to the staffroom regularly to discuss matters of school policy or to inform herself about an individual pupil's welfare. However, in this particular environment of the staffroom, the interchange of opinions and ideas did not encourage innovation but, on the contrary, reinforced the existing consensus which favoured the grammar-school ethos. Mr Ellis, whose job as an advisory teacher (English), covering 38 schools, made him particularly well-qualified to comment on one positive aspect of the regime: 'This is one of the few schools I like to teach in, maybe it is because of Ms Grey's caring and professional approach.' However, not all the staff were complacent about what they considered to be a 'regressive' school ethos that ignored the positive aims of comprehensivisation. Some younger members of staff recognised the rift this 'old-fashioned' way of conducting school affairs caused between the pupils and the teachers, as one member of staff explained: 'There is a lot of distrust between the girls and the staff . . . they each live in different worlds. You often hear the word 'snob' in the corridors when the girls refer to the teachers' (Ms Land: Geography teacher).

The resistance to change at St Theresa's brought about not only the alienation of pupils but also an estrangement between staff and parents, as one teacher observed: 'There is a problem of misunderstanding between parents and teachers at St Theresa's. It stems from different ideas that each have of the school and what to expect from the school' (Ms James: English teacher).

3 The curriculum and teaching methods

In 1984, seven years after the 1976 comprehensive reorganisation of the educational system, there was little evidence at St Theresa's of any willingness to compromise the heavy academic emphasis of the curriculum and traditional teaching methods of the past. Whereas the high-ability girls received much attention from the staff, who enjoyed the challenge of their presence, the lower-ability pupils were less fortunate. Streaming, which ensured the hierarchical separation of low- from high-ability pupils, reinforced a divisive system of education that was the hallmark of St Theresa's.

In sharp contrast to what was available to the more able pupils, academic concessions to the less able were limited. The lessons of Band 3 pupils throughout the school were often observed to be educationally unproductive and difficult to teach. Rather than re-evaluate the situation and in particular the teacher's approach to difficult classes, the school's immediate reaction was to withdraw academic privilege, as the following example shows. The head of the Modern Language department explained that the second- and third-year pupils were no longer to be taught French. Her reason was as follows: 'because of the disruptive behaviour of the pupils. They just cannot concentrate during listening work.'

A decision such as this had serious repercussions for the pupils concerned who were being denied access, without appeal, to learning an important foreign language so early in their secondary career. This decision was made on the basis of one teacher's evaluation, the truth of which was never questioned.

The school's policy with regard to homework also reflected its bias towards the more academically inclined. In the 'top' ability groups homework was set for each lesson. In contrast, homework for the lower-ability sets was given less regularly, which was, as outlined in the Quinquennial Review, 'when practical and necessary or to complete work already begun in the class' (p. 127).

If an academic future for a pupil was not possible then the school's policy was to move to the other extreme and react by withdrawal from lessons, substituting special education or remedial classes for normal lessons. Non-academic courses were also set up mainly for the benefit of the less able. These courses – Personal and Social Education, Looking Forward, Clerical and Office Skills – were ill conceived, poorly organised and badly staffed, as Ms Wallace, a teacher committed to developing the Looking Forward programme explained: 'There is insufficient time to develop the course and limited opportunity to discuss the course with other staff.'

The Quinquennial Review did remark that in general, at St Theresa's: 'The curriculum focuses too much on academic work and not enough on practical sessions' (p. 25).

However, the timetabling priority of these practical sessions was such that they were not accessible to the more able pupils. Even the less academic (albeit 'female-centred') subject options such as Child Development and Office Skills were not available to girls who were engaged in the academic curriculum. Personal and Social Education which was a 'pastoral' course scheduled for everyone, was viewed as 'prep' time by the more academic, and permission not to attend was common.

It was apparent that the school's policy was to present the less academic option as the solution, rather than adapting and improving the teaching and learning within the mainstream, exam-orientated curriculum for the less academic pupil. In the Quinquennial Review, the headmistress justifies this approach in the following way: 'The course begins to fulfil a need for the less academic option choices as many of the comprehensive pupils seem under intense pressure and are finding it difficult to cope' (p. 96).

However, during the several months that I spent at St Theresa's it was apparent that these non-academic, practical sessions were not conceived in the best interests of the pupils concerned. They were in effect no more than 'containment periods', for what were perceived to be 'difficult' and 'disruptive' girls. Those defined as less able were separated off from the others, put into classrooms and supervised minimally. In these lessons they learned little or nothing, as hardly anything was taught, although these girls did receive an internal school certificate for completion of a minimum course requirement.

Resources allocated to these more practical sessions were clearly limited. The secondary status of these courses meant that the budget allowance was minimal, there were no rooms allocated for these subjects and there were no qualified staff to teach them. Teachers who were 'free' were sent to supervise or teach these classes. I was readily allowed access to these lesson times for interviewing purposes. On several occasions I was asked to sit with the pupils and supervise the session as no one else was available. I was given the following advice: 'Just talk to them. They feel no one cares. They think school is against them and everything is against them. In general they feel the authority of the school weighs down on them' (Ms Wallace: English teacher and head of Careers).

Although they had been relegated to the 'educational dustbin' at St Theresa's, there was no evidence to suggest that these girls were incapable of learning. Despite being clearly alienated from the staff, I found them articulate, keen and interested. They willingly participated in my research, and despite warnings from the staff to the contrary, they had their own opinions on political and social issues.

4 Discipline and control

On matters of discipline Ms Grey had a firm and active policy, which was supported by the staff. It was an aspect of St Theresa's regime that was of central concern. In the Quinquennial Review the largest section was devoted to the school's policy on matters of discipline and control. In the daily events of the school this emphasis on discipline was evident. The school office was a busy place, full of parents and girls, many of whom were awaiting disciplinary procedures. A central reception area of the school housed a bench where offending girls sat in punishment.

In sharp contrast to the attitude at St Hilda's, truancy was dealt with uncompromisingly. Parents were summoned immediately to discuss the matter with Ms Grey and the Education Welfare Officer. While I was at St Theresa's there were several cases of truancy, one of which was going to court. Other forms of disciplinary procedures included a rigid detention policy, and girls were often put 'on report', rather than being suspended. The school also had an abundance of rules for the girls to comply with; ignorance was no excuse for non-adherence.

It was evident that the formidable regime with regard to discipline was associated with what was regarded as the 'new and difficult intake', most of whom were black. This was clearly stated in the Quinquennial Review by Ms Masters, the head of Pastoral Care: 'The all-ability intake has brought a much greater proportion of girls whose behaviour has given serious cause for concern' (p. 19). Ms Grey exerted a powerful control over discipline problems in her school, as the following example illustrates.

Elderly residents from a nearby (all white) council estate complained to the school that they were being 'harassed' by gangs of black girls. Although this claim was never substantiated (there was a tuck shop on the estate that the girls frequented, much to the annoyance of the local residents), Ms Grey responded by giving the lower school and those classes in the upper school with a notorious reputation for being difficult, detention for a week. This blanket action, which the uninvolved girls found unwarranted, caused much resentment and did little to resolve the situation. It created an undercurrent of hostility and distrust between the staff and the pupils, and both parties increasingly regarded the other with suspicion.

The outcome of the overtly disciplinarian and punitive approach of the school toward the 'all-ability intake' was to reinforce the system of 'containment' which was already evident in the non-academic and academic dichotomy of the curriculum.

5 Multi-racial education

Unlike Mr Madden, Ms Grey was more astute when it came to matters that reflected on the school's 'good reputation'. This was illustrated in Ms Grey's approach to MRE in her school. Both in interviews and in the Quinquennial Review she paid much lip-service to the ILEA's policy of MRE. Ms Grey told me of a Church of England project that was to be undertaken in the school. The project's aim was to investigate the 'successful' destinations of young black women who had attended the school during the last ten years. Ms Grey was acutely aware of how to manipulate the political rhetoric that surrounded the issue of race in schools to serve her own interests. In sharp contrast to her obvious feelings about the decline in the school's standards with the introduction of a more multi-racial intake, she said about the project: 'It is a worthy and positive cause. It aims to counteract negative stereotypes of West Indians. It is very important that the successful stories are told.'

Ms Grey confirmed her support of MRE in the Quinquennial Review as follows: 'We need to find time to explore a number of cross-curricular issues, in particular our policy for multi-ethnic education and our methods and assessment of pupils in line with recent ILEA initatives' (p. 7).

However, in spite of these statements there was no evidence at St Theresa's that MRE was an active priority in the way Ms Grey suggested. On the contrary, the staff in general were uninformed and unconcerned about the issue. For example, when the sixth form mistress and senior member of staff, Ms Carter, was asked about the performance and aspirations of her black female pupils she replied, 'To tell you the truth I've never given it much thought.'

6 Single-sex status[7]

An aspect of St Theresa's that contributed to the particular climate of the school was the fact that it retained its single-sex status after comprehensivisation. Some staff felt that the school benefited from being exclusively for girls:

It is important that this is a single-sex school. Girls are more assured and confident in an all-girls atmosphere. But, as we know, schools cannot make up for what goes on in the outside world. Ultimately there is little a school can do to change sexism, and, I should point out, sexism can still exist in an all-girls' school.

(Ms Bernard: Music teacher)

Other teachers, however, felt it to be a definite drawback, as Ms Tinker, a Science teacher, explained:

I was surprised when I came here how difficult girls are. I pre-ferred teaching at Bishop John [large all boys' comprehensive nearby]. The boys were better behaved. The girls are brasher here. There is such a strong subculture among them that you can't get through to them. People talk about Bishop John, its reputation and all, but I felt there was a lot more staff support there and it was a lot more rewarding to teach.

There was evidence at St Theresa's to suggest that the all-girls learning environment was, on the whole, beneficial. Unlike their counterparts at St Hilda's, the girls were more likely to do tradition-ally male-defined subjects (for example, sciences were popular) and did not have to contend with their marginalisation in the classroom.

At St Theresa's it did appear that the satisfactory performance of the Band 1 girls could be related to the fact that they were in an all-female learning environment; however, being in an all-girls school did not account for the comparatively unsatisfactory perfor-mance of the less able pupils. This suggests that the discrepancy in educational performance between high-ability and low-ability girls at St Theresa's was due to other factors than the single-sex nature of the school.

Thus, in summing up, it was found that at St Theresa's, whereas the high-ability girls, regardless of social class, fared well within the grammar-school ethos of the school, the lower-ability pupils experi-enced five years of what can only be described as 'custodial edu-cation'. These lower-ability girls, who were defined as 'difficult', were not only subject to rigid rules and restrictions, but were further 'contained' by a system of streaming that ensured their separation and placement into non-academic courses, withdrawal from normal class, or second-rate attention in their academic lessons. This duality in treatment between the high-ability and low-ability girls was reflec-ted in the notable discrepancy that existed in the examination results of those classified as able and those defined as less able to cope with academic work. Black girls fared poorly in this inherently inequitable regime, not least because the method of recruitment ensured that a disproportionate number of them entered the school in the lower-ability grades.

CONCLUSION: CAN SCHOOLS COMPENSATE FOR SOCIETY?[8]

Because examination results impinge dramatically on career destinations, the quality of a pupil's performance is a significant determinant. My findings did suggest that, with regard to examination results, the school that an individual pupil attended did make a difference. The difference I observed between St Hilda's on the one hand, with its record of academic mediocrity, and St Theresa's on the other, with its apparent selective regime, could be attributed to an overall difference in school leadership and hence ethos. A consideration of this evidence could suggest that a school in isolation can, if it is well run, affect pupil outcome. Indeed this is a proposition put forward by Rutter et al. (1979), who conclude: 'Schools can do much to foster good behaviour and attainments and that even in a disadvantaged area, schools can be a force for the good' (p. 205).

Although schools clearly do make a difference, it is quite another thing to suggest that schools can compensate for society, as Rutter et al. seem to suggest. Micro-studies of the school, such as those of Rutter and Mortimore, are in danger of ignoring the wider social and economic forces that affect the school's independence as a social institution.

My general conclusion must therefore be that, while a great deal can be discovered about more effective teaching and learning from studies such as the one presented here, such research by no means offers a solution to the endemic problem of inequality that is an integral feature of schools in British society. In order to arrive at a more productive analysis of the way in which wider social influences impinge on the maintenance of social inequality, we need to turn to a more detailed evaluation of schooling in Britain in terms of its effects on occupational choice.

Chapter 4

Life in the classroom

Of the many theoretical perspectives that have contributed to the debate on the nature of the educational experience, two ideological camps are distinguishable. On the one hand there are those that emphasise the institutional level, the structure, operation and functions of schooling; on the other, there are those that find analysis at the personal interactive level more important. These theorists, who emphasise the inner workings of the classroom, focus in particular on the relationships between teacher and pupil.

Attempts to describe the black educational experience have been characterised, in the main, by research designs ideologically disposed towards the latter perspective, with early studies investigating the causes and effects of negative black self-esteem (Milner 1975, 1983; Coard 1971). Employing the notion of the self-fulfilling prophecy and the mechanism of labelling, these studies focused on the effect a teacher might have on a pupil's own self-image.

A central proposition of such research is that pupils tend to perform as well or as badly as their teachers expect. The teacher's prediction of a pupil's behaviour, it is suggested, is communicated to them, frequently in unintended ways, influencing the actual behaviour that follows. Thus it is only logical to assume that if teachers hold stereotyped opinions and expectations of black children, this may lead to different teaching techniques and classroom treatment, which works to the detriment of these children's education.

Indeed, it was not uncommon to find teachers expressing openly their misgivings about the intellectual capabilities of the black girls in their care. During informal conversation and formal interviews that I had with them, 75 per cent of the teachers in the study made at least one negative comment about the black girls they taught. I was told by one fifth-year teacher and careers mistress that: 'Most of these girls will never succeed . . . they are just unable to remember, the girls just can't make it at this level ['O' level and CSE], never mind what is demanded in higher education. There is what I call "brain death" among them . . . unable to think for themselves.' With statements such as these, teachers provide easy targets, offering tangible and powerful evidence against themselves. It is not surprising, therefore, that they are assumed by many social commentators to be the central link in the transmission of social and racial inequality. This is a convenient and obvious causal assumption to make. However, while the evidence presented in this chapter does suggest that teachers do have interpretative schemes upon which they make predictions concerning pupil ability, the findings of this study do not uphold the notion of the self-fulfilling prophecy as a central explanation for black underachievement.

THE PUPIL PERSPECTIVE: A CHALLENGE TO THE SELF-FULFILLING PROPHECY

There appeared to be two major reasons why the self-fulfilling prophecy failed to provide an adequate understanding of the observed classroom process. Firstly, there was nothing in the evidence to suggest that teachers were successful in eroding black female self-esteem. Secondly, the findings do not show that teachers transmitted their apparent negative expectations to the black pupils they teach. According to the logic of the self-fulfilling prophecy, these two aspects of the labelling process are fundamental to its successful operation.

There was no indication that young black women had negative feelings about being black or female. The girls greatly valued their cultural and racial identity. Of young black women, in answer to the question 'Who is the person you most admire?', 48 per cent indicated that this person was herself.[1] Furthermore, when the qualities of the person each pupil indicated as the person they most admired were analysed it was found that 55 per cent of the black women had chosen a person who was black, as did 50 per cent of the young black men. The young black women also frequently chose a female person as 'the person they most admired' (11 per cent chose their mother, 5 per cent a female relative, 9 per cent a female historical figure).

There was also little evidence of young black females suffering psychological damage from being 'put down' as a consequence of their teachers' negative evaluations of them. Clearly the girls did not accept the negative evaluations of themselves and their academic abilities, as the following example shows. Ms Wallace, when describing a predominantly black fifth-year class designated as of 'low ability', said: 'These girls have absolutely no motivation. They feel you are here to think for them.' Yet these same girls said of their teachers: 'They hold you back. Teachers always put you down, then they say, 'You can't manage. . . . ' (Dianne: aged 16); 'When you come you sit a test and then after that they never give you a chance to prove yourself' (Tony: aged 16).

The young black women, when interviewed, were aware of their teachers' negative feelings towards them:

> You feel the discrimination, they try to hide it but you can see through it. They try to say, 'We're all equal', but you can tell: they talk to you more simply.
>
> (Maureen: aged 16)

> Some teachers show that they wouldn't like to teach you. I feel this attitude is absolutely wrong. They are paid to teach pupils, not to pick and choose who they would like to teach.
>
> (Karen: aged 17)

Although the girls were resentful of these attitudes, there was little evidence that they were psychologically undermined by this differential treatment. On the contrary, the girls often challenged these assumptions about their ability and confronted the situation openly, as this student's account reveals:

> My maths teacher really treat us differently. One day I was stuck on a question, I called him over he said, 'Oh, you know how to do this. . . . ' Afterwards this white girl which he likes quite a lot, she was on the same question as me, she did not understand it then he really did explain it to her and he said, 'Selma you can listen now if you want to'. Then I said, 'Never mind'. He never tells her off. She goes and talks to the other pupils but when I get up he starts to shout at me . . . then I say, 'Why don't you tell her'. He always picks on mostly all the black girls. [sic]
>
> (Selma: aged 16)

An outcome of this pupil awareness of negative teacher evaluations of them was that black children refuse to present their real selves in school. It was apparent that the black girls would avoid asking for help, as Selma did in the example above. The girls would only approach certain members of staff known to be compliant, or only participate keenly in certain lessons taught by such sympathetic teachers. They would also avoid choosing certain subjects if the teacher was recognised as being difficult, as this statement made by a fifth-year pupil at St Theresa's shows: 'I like English, but I know Mrs Webster hates me. I'll just end up failing. No one wants to do English because of Mrs Webster' (Angela: aged 16).

It was a fact that in many cases the girls' academic energies were often diverted to strategies aimed at avoiding unpleasant scenarios within the school environment, rather than in the activity of learning.

If the explanation for the way in which teachers affect pupil performance does not lie within an understanding of the notion of the self-fulfilling prophecy, the question remains as to how exactly does teacher–pupil interaction function to disadvantage the black child? The evidence seemed to suggest that the process of discrimination operated by means of the teachers' access to physical and material resources, restrictions to which would result in the curtailment of opportunities. Clearly teachers do have the power to effect changes and limit or enhance pupil opportunity. As an outcome of their power within the institutional infrastructure teachers are in a position to enforce their prejudices by restricting access to information and educational resources. The positive pupil perspective, which has been persistently overlooked in the trend to highlight black negative self-esteem, brings to the fore the importance of power and control in the classroom.

RACISM AND REACTION: A TEACHER TYPOLOGY

The findings of this study revealed many shades of teacher reaction to the race, gender and social class of their pupils (see also Mac an Ghaill 1988). In the following pages I attempt to analyse some of the attitudinal characteristics I found among staff in the schools, and assess the outcome of their specific beliefs and values on the black female pupils in their classrooms. Five general teacher responses were identified. These were grouped as follows: (1) the 'Overt Racists', (2) the 'Christians', (3) the 'Crusaders', (4) the 'Liberal Chauvinists' and (5) the 'Black Teacher'.

1 The 'Overt Racists'

As high a proportion as 33 per cent of teachers interviewed in the study held what can only be described as overtly racist opinions. It appeared that at the 'grass-roots' level of the staffroom, many teachers remained untouched by the vigorous anti-racist debates and campaigns that were taking place around them.[2] In spite of attempts to inform them to the contrary, these teachers held fast to their convictions as to the intellectual and cultural inferiority of their black pupils, often expressing open resentment at their presence in their country and their school.

Examples of overt racist sentiment and practice were not always confined to isolated incidents or statements, but were often the consequence of long-standing, bitter feuds between certain members of staff and pupils, situations fuelled by racist action and pupil reaction.

Mr Davidson was a young History teacher who derived a definite pleasure from taunting the black pupils, particularly the boys. One black male pupil reported the following incident, apparently one of many, in confidence:

> Mr Davidson called me a wog. Me and my friend we turned round and saw Davidson looking at us and then he said get inside. He also said, 'Don't drop peanuts or coconuts on the floor', the peanuts belonged to a white boy behind him. But Davidson said nothing to him. After school he kept me and some other black kids. [sic]
>
> (Davis: aged 16: aspiration, armed forces)

Mr Davidson's obvious dislike of black pupils was not confined to verbal abuse of black males. Females were not immune from his disdain, which I discovered to my cost, when I had a door knowingly and sadistically slammed in my face. Neither was his overt racism hidden from the other members of staff, many of whom harboured similar sentiments but were less forthcoming about them. Mr Davidson openly voiced his disapproval of the Multi-Racial Working Party, announcing his intention to boycott the meetings. He also claimed, in his capacity as History teacher, that:

> African history is so boring. . . . I had to do it at college, it was part of the course. Old civilisations are boring and the discussion of slavery is monotonous in school teaching . . . it has no bearing on anything.

The opinions and actions of Davidson were extreme. But how far can such attitudes be dismissed as exceptions to the rule and isolated incidents, as extreme cases so often are? While Davidson's racist behaviour was more overt than that displayed by others, incidents of overt racism were by no means an exceptional occurrence. Many members of staff deeply resented the presence of black pupils in their school and often articulated this point of view.

The school secretary, Ms Simpson, had a reputation that preceded her. The girls in her school constantly complained of the way she reacted towards them: keeping their parents waiting, not answering politely, and generally being as unhelpful as possible. There is always the matter of character misrepresentation in such reports and I was careful not to believe everything I was told. However, I witnessed an incident in the corridor that confirmed the girls' reports to me of her negative attitudes towards them.

During a class change-over, at the end of a period, Ms Simpson pushed past me, making her way angrily towards a group of black girls walking slowly and chatting away loudly among themselves. Obviously enraged, she shouted loudly: 'WILL YOU STOP THAT AT ONCE! . . . Honestly, the way you people conduct yourself you wouldn't think you were part of civilisation!'

As she turned and walked towards me again, she muttered: 'I just don't know, things were so different before *they* came . . . honestly. . . . ' Almost bumping into me she agitatedly added: 'Oh, get out of my way' (and then rushed off).

Ms Bland, an Art teacher for many years, explained how she felt about her black pupils:

> I'm fed up with them. Everyone is fed up . . . only they won't say it. They are so loud and inconsiderate. . . . They are always talking about being black, chip on the shoulder, haven't met one who hasn't. . . . Why can't people be people. Everyone's so over-sensitive nowadays!
>
> All this about golliwogs, for instance, banning golliwogs! I ask you. I love my golly, and you tell me what is wrong with that. Imagine, in Brixton they wanted to put up black angels, did you hear? Black angels, how ridiculous! Why give them a race? Angels are angels, they have always been white, why change now? It's only going to make things worse, my dear . . . all this advice. . . . Yes, that ILEA business . . . telling us what to think. . . . Well, my

dear I honestly feel at times to give up my job . . . after all these years forced to give up my job, imagine?

Sister Margarita, a nun and first-year head at St Hilda's, had a reputation both in the school and in the wider community (young mothers at the local youth centre made reference to her attitude), for not only being a difficult and often unpleasant, humourless person (she was *very* strict), but also, as one colleague called her, 'a bit of a bigot'. Her particular attitude was one that was characterised by ignorance and intolerance, as the following incidents illustrate.

Sister Margarita was called to interview some prospective parents to the school. However, the school secretary on delivering the message that they were on their way up, also whispered to her that they were 'black'. Sister Margarita immediately became agitated and said to the secretary, 'I'm busy, tell them to wait'. Eventually, after some time, she did go. However, when she returned she exclaimed, surprised, to several colleagues, 'Do you know he was a doctor . . . a black doctor!' Sister Margarita's limited racist perceptions had, in this instance, received a jolt.

Even though Sister Margarita herself was humourless and stern, her ignorance often caused amusement. When the Education Officer of the borough came to the school, Sister Margarita was taken aback when he, Mr Henry, who was himself black, struck up a conversation with her about a mutual acquaintance, another nun. Sister was visibly surprised by the connection, and to the amusement of many of the staff spoke clearly and loudly to Mr Henry as if she were speaking to a 'foreigner' who could not understand English.

'Amusing' though Sister Margarita's naïve and ignorant attitudes might be, she often displayed the depth of her convictions, making what she felt to be logical assumptions about the black children, over whom she had considerable authority. For example, during a staff-room conversation about the possibility of a school sports day, Sister Margarita expressed her concern, saying: 'You can't have a sports day, things just wouldn't be fair, all the blacks would win all the prizes and that would cause only trouble.' This prompted a sharp reply from a colleague, who said, 'So it's all right if all the whites win!'

The existence of several studies that have also found overt forms of racism prevalent among teachers in schools suggest that the presence of this form of racism is more widespread than is often recognised (DES 1985; Wright, in Eggleston *et al*. 1986, 1987). Apart from the situations mentioned so far, the passing of references to assumed inherent characteristics of black students was often to be heard in the staffroom and openly stated to me. For example, one pleasant and helpful young male teacher (he was doing an MA in Education) warned, 'You have to watch them [that is, black girls], they can be sly.' Another explained, 'They are angry and frustrated with their lot, and can get very hostile when they get into a group.'

The evidence suggests that the work of the scientific racists has to a significant degree permeated normative thought and belief about the inherent inferiority and superiority of the various races and cultures. People do make, and find it necessary to make, generalisations about people from limited information in everyday life. However, the type of assumptions being made by certain members of staff about black pupils were clearly negative and thus had consequences for the black student.

2 The 'Christians'

The 'Christians' were a distinctive group who lived up to their name. These teachers were identifiable by their capacity for compassion towards and conviction about the equality of their black brothers and sisters.[3] The particular concept of equality employed by the 'Christians' led to a consensus that, in general, characterised this attitude: that is, the 'colour-blind' approach to the education of the black child. What guided this approach was the philosophy that 'We are all the same . . . there are no differences, *and there are no problems'*: a celebration of 'sameness'. As one teacher pointed out, 'We see them as pupils first, not if they are black or white.'

The following extract from St Hilda's school newsletter, written by the headmaster, Mr Madden, exemplifies this 'Christian' orientation to the black presence in British schools.[4] He writes:

Headmaster's Letter to Parents: Spring Mid-Term 1984

Dear parents,

Multi-Ethnic Education

I am convinced that you like me, wonder what this is all about? What are these words, ethnic, racialism, discrimination, minorities, equal opportunities, the British Movement and the National Front, etc. etc. and etc.? White parents and black parents pride themselves on treating all children, whatever the colour, in the fairest way possible. After all we are all Catholic men and women and we all know the story of the Good Samaritan in the Gospels where the foreign visitor took great care of his enemy, the badly injured Jewish traveller. . . . I could go on extolling our virtues but it would be incorrect.

Today in our schools, in our neighbourhood, in the place where we work, in the pubs, discotheques and everywhere we go, we will have children and adults who are not white and who may have different ideas about many different aspects of life, etc. to which they are fully entitled.

I think the general attitude from white people at best is to tolerate them and their differences although we really like charming French accents or chic Italian-style shoes. To be honest with ourselves we haven't really tried to come to terms with these black children and adults and all you have to do is to look around the school or perhaps look at the number of black teenagers who are unemployed. . . .

This extract illustrates not only the 'well-intentioned' nature of this ideological perspective, but it also highlights the gulf of experience that exists between the white staff and the black pupil: a 'them-and-us' situation mediated by the belief in tolerance and understanding as a solution to the endemic problem of racial discrimination.

However, this attitude in itself, although limiting, was not necessarily harmful to the pupils. What gave this particular 'Christian' orientation its negative impact was the reaction it engendered from the teachers to any form of positive action that aimed to redress racial discrimination. At St Hilda's, for example, the setting-up of a Multi-Racial Working Party was objected to on the grounds of a general consensus that all pupils were treated equally in the school and that therefore there was no racial discrimination, in spite of evidence to the contrary.

An example of this general attitude was illustrated in a staff meeting at St Hilda's, where a report submitted by the MRE Working Party[5] led to a discussion of race and racism in the school. In the meeting there was a great deal of hostility towards the suggestion that there was any form or practice of racism at St Hilda's. When the representatives of the school's Working Party outlined their draft statement on how racism manifests itself in the school and how it should be tackled, the statement was met by non-response, with many members of the staff choosing not to participate in the discussion.

The staff's negative response to the Working Party's suggestions was largely directed towards the ILEA and what was considered to be its interfering insistence that racism is a problem for schools in London. They articulated their resentment:

> We are fair here, I think this is an unwelcome imposition from the ILEA. I believe we would have come round to a discussion of the matter in our own time. . . . I don't feel we needed to be told. I think we are being pushed . . .
>
> (Mr Gavin: Mathematics teacher, St Hilda's)

> What do they [the ILEA] mean by black? They try to give us their ideas of what black is. . . . I think it is a bit of a cheek really. Don't you? Well, it's all well and good but it's a lot of talk, they don't give us much back-up or help, do they?
>
> (Ms Prime: French mistress, St Hilda's)

> Think it's down to this . . . the authority has told us we must do something so we must not quibble with the authority, we must be seen to be doing something.
>
> (Mr Sutton: head of the fifth year and D & T teacher)

The resentment stemmed from the strong belief that racism was not present in the school nor was cultural diversity an issue they needed to address, as several of the staff explained:

> I really don't think we are as affected as other schools. We are all Christians here. That is our culture, and our way of life, black and white, I really can't see that there has been a spread of any other different culture.
>
> (Ms Cole: Religious and General Studies teacher)

> We don't need to know where they come from . . . colour is not important. I'm not interested in people's backgrounds, I treat everyone by their own worth as individuals.
>
> (Mr Simpson: head of the third year and History teacher)

> There is no need to go out of your way to find out information about them. It could be regarded as prying, but if they offer information that is another thing.
>
> (Ms Phillips: head of English)

The conclusion to this discussion of race in the staff meeting was an interesting one. It was decided that there was no need for guidelines or disciplinary action for racist behaviour in the classroom. It was felt that dealing with such issues was an individual matter. There was also a strong feeling among the staff that they did not need to be told how to conduct their internal affairs, not only because that was tantamount to interference, but also, as one teacher explained, because it could lead to problems when, as they agreed, there were none:

> By talking about racism, making it an issue, coloured pupils can get aggressive. I've seen it at St Joan's . . . the atmosphere is so tense. You feel threatened just going in there. Teachers have been attacked there, terrorised, I've heard. I don't want that here, not here. We have a happy and healthy atmosphere here.
>
> (Ms Cole: Religious and General Studies teacher)

The refusal to recognise the existence of racism and the effect that this oversight might have on black pupils can again be illustrated by the response of Mr Madden, the headmaster of St Hilda's, to my application to undertake to do research in his school. Mr Madden was very keen and interested about my wanting to do research in his school, and in particular my emphasis on black girls. He explained:

> I suppose you know and indeed we are very proud that we have several black girls here doing very well . . . we are pleased about that. It is good that you are here. I understand that there is a lot of interest in the performance of black girls. As you will see we are doing fine, very well. There is very little that I can tell you as everything is fine, as it should be, may I say. You know we don't make special cases and I am sure when it comes down to it that is why they do so well.

However, the truth was far from Mr Madden's claims. While there were several black girls in the top achievement stream of the school, as he had said, these girls did not owe their placement in this Band 1 stream to the policy of non-recognition upheld by the headmaster and his staff. The educational achievements of the black girls in the school were in spite of and not because of the schooling they received. During my months of fieldwork, as the final examinations of the fifth year became imminent, it became clear that all was not well with the black girls in the top stream, as Anita, one of these girls, explained:

I hate streaming, I hate it, miss, I wish they never had it. [Anita explained that she felt that 'they' (the school) did not care about her or others like her, that all the school wanted was for them to be seen to be doing well.] They's just want to be looking good . . . . They keep on and on at you . . . you must do well, you gotta do well . . . so much all the time I tell you. I so fed up. . . . They expect so much from you.

Anita was almost in tears when she described the pressure she was under with the exams coming up, and said, 'They think it so easy, miss, they think it so easy, you know.'

The teachers did have high expectations of their Band 1 pupils, but the evidence suggested that at the same time there was a limited amount of support and educational preparation for these pupils.[6] In spite of the girls' obvious need for assistance during this crucial time of their educational career,[7] the teachers remained steadfast in their belief that no special case should be made as all pupils were held to be the same.

The following statement by Ms Phillips, an English teacher, illustrates the rationale that resulted in this 'Christian', colour-blind attitude among the staff:

You can see that Anita is very good at her work. She and the others are all bright but they will get together and talk. . . . Well, I don't want to say anything for peace sake, you know. . . . They can be so disruptive and then I'll have a situation on my hands.' It's better not to say anything, at least that has been my experience. I don't want to rock the boat, as it were, you know. . . . They seem to manage quite well in their own way.

For 'peace sake' Ms Phillips did not want to push the girls academically by insisting on their concentration and participation. She was satisfied to leave the girls to their own devices even though she was aware of their potential. Often Ms Phillips' lessons were unruly and disorganised; on the whole difficult learning forums for the pupils. The colour-blind approach of this teacher was useful neither to the staff nor to the pupils and, as this example showed, clearly jeopardised the educational outcome for all concerned.

Furthermore, the unwillingness to take a strong stand on educational issues concerning the black child for fear of 'rocking the boat', a basic characteristic of the 'Christian' attitude, had the effect of both misleading and misinforming black parents about the progress of their children, as the following example illustrates. Marion's mother had been under the impression that her daughter's progress at school was satisfactory. Marion's reports all indicated that she was working well – 'Progress good' was what was written in the annual reports. Ms Dale, Marion's mother, was therefore very surprised when she was called to the school for a formal meeting to discuss Marion's poor levels of attainment.

> I thought she doing OK. They said she doing good, and doing good is doing good, not so? But now the teacher say I must understand that doing good is a relative thing. Marion was doing good for Marion, not just doing good.

Ms Dale felt that she had been misled about her daughter's progress, because, as it transpired, the teacher concerned did not want to disappoint her black pupil. The effect of this teacher's 'kindness' was not only upsetting for both Marion and her parents, it was also detrimental to her long-term progress. Marion was unprepared for her exams and eventually had to give up two subjects in order that she might be able to cope with the rest of her work.

This form of patronage was not an isolated incident. Other cases occurred where, in order to avoid disappointment or to encourage their black pupils, teachers were found to be giving the wrong impression of a child's progress. In Tony's case this was a particularly misplaced gesture by the teachers concerned.

Tony was a young black woman who had been in care most of her life. To encourage her the staff at St Theresa's had, as in the case of Marion, given the impression in her school reports that her progress had been good. Eventually this strategy began to have negative consequences and the head of year had to ring up the home Tony was at and tell them, much to their surprise, that her progress was not as had been thought and she was in need of some strong re-evaluation in order to rectify the situation with regard to her future.

The evidence was clear, the 'Christian' approach, despite its benevolent and passive characteristics, can have negative consequences for black pupils. By adopting a 'colour-blind' perspective, the staff and the schools concerned created an atmosphere where ignorance and fear remained unchallenged. Any reference to colour was, among the 'Christians', an accepted taboo, as its very mention implied that there existed racial differences.

3 The 'Crusaders'

In contrast to the 'Christians', the 'Crusaders' were prepared to acknowledge that racism was present within educational establishments. This group of teachers held strong beliefs that this racism among their colleagues and the pupils they taught should be challenged. These teachers were therefore dedicated to action; that is, action of a political sort and indeed action as sanctioned and prescribed by the ILEA.

Comparatively, the 'Crusaders' were few in number; just 2 per cent of the teachers in the study lived up to the reputation as active 'anti-racist campaigners'. The distinctive characteristics of the 'Crusaders' were their colour (white), their youth and their commitment to their cause. This latter aspect that in particular identified this group, the commitment to their cause, was characterised by a strategy that sought to 'educate' colleagues into the wrongs of the past and the injustices of the present. Ms Wallace, a teacher at St Theresa's, shared her sweeping radical views when she explained enthusiastically:

> What we need to do is eradicate, get rid of this white elitist education we have, leave it behind, I ask you what relevance is Shakespeare nowadays? That goes for everyone, not just for the black kids.

Not surprisingly, in view of the reaction of the majority of teachers to the issue of race (already discussed), together with their often dogmatic approach, the 'Crusaders' found little sympathy for their cause among their colleagues. The experiences of Rachel Spencer, a young Drama teacher at St Hilda's, illustrates the frustrations and futility of the often over-zealous and misguided anti-racist campaign that was the hallmark of the 'Crusaders'.

In accordance with the guidelines of the ILEA's directives on anti-racism (ILEA 1983), Ms Spencer had been engaged for several months in the difficult (but voluntary) task of setting up a Multi-Racial Working Party in her school, St Hilda's. One day, totally exasperated with her struggle, she explained: 'We are *breaking* ILEA policy, actually going against it by not doing anything positive. We *must* do something.' She had come up against several obstacles in her attempts to establish the Working Party, not least because of the headmaster's own objections. His dissent was grounded in his feeling that the Working Party was an intrusion and a violation of the school's private affairs by an outside body, the ILEA, mediated by Ms Spencer. Mr Madden also felt, like many others, that racism was not an issue. As Spencer explained, her campaign was frustrated at every turn:

> Madden has no interest in working parties . . . so he does not attend, not even to give any moral support. So you can imagine this lazy lot do not bother to attend, maybe one or two out of how many of us? Thirty or so? Well, I suppose there are no promotional prospects in attending . . . so why bother? No one's going to stay on till 5.30 when they can go home at 4.00 if they don't have to, are they? Even at lunch-time there is a problem. I'm really fed up, dealing with people that just don't care. Yesterday I wanted to call a meeting at lunch but because some of them wanted to play football they said I can't have it at lunch. Everyone moans, they can't come at that time or at this time. They don't seem to understand that it is school policy I am talking about. No one has shown any interest in that plan of mine to speak to the fifth and fourth years. . . . You won't believe this, Madden actually said that I cannot go to the meeting that I arranged with Mr Bacchus [Borough MRE inspector]. Guess his excuse? There is no one to cover for my lesson. . . . A bit weak, I think.

Ms Spencer was not the only member of staff at St Hilda's to experience the frustrations produced by the apathy of colleagues. Mr Mahon, in a final effort to arouse some support for the MRE Working Party and its anti-racist campaign, had this to say:

> What we should do is send a report to the inspectorate saying 'we find no racism here and that we have resolved all our problems about racism', that will get them going. What a laugh the authority will have. This will be a miracle school, the only one in London to have eradicated racism.

While Rachel Spencer saw her colleagues as suspicious, backward and inherently prejudiced, they on the other hand regarded her and the other committed anti-racist campaigners in a not too serious light, as somewhat eccentric and going through a 'phase', a bit of a nuisance. Ms Spencer was aware of how she was being patronised by her fellow teachers:

> They see me as a tizzy [sic] young woman with a bee in my bonnet about this race thing, who gets upset easily. They try to put you

down, Mr Madden is always saying things like 'Don't worry, dear
. . . . Don't get upset, dear'.

Making them less threatening by evaluating them as harmless 'radi-
cals' was a way some members of staff at St Hilda's had developed to
deal with the often uncompromising demands of the 'Crusaders'. For
example, it was not uncommon to find some teachers making fun of
their colleagues on the basis of their dress, appearance, age or sex, as
this teacher explained:

> No one takes Rachel seriously. She gives the impression of being
> so disorganised and inefficient, but I suppose she gets there in the
> end. I want to tell her what I think, well what we all think, but I
> haven't got the heart, just look at what she has got on today! She
> tries so hard I suppose I just can't. It is the image one gives that
> achieves results. It is so important, even though Rachel, she is
> doing things, people do not see her directions.
>
> (Ms Cole: Religious and General Studies teacher)

There was little doubt that the 'Crusaders' were dedicated to the
cause of anti-racism: however, their actions were not always in the
best interests of the black pupils in their care. Often, because of the
futility and frustrations of their actions, a great deal of the 'Crusaders',
teaching energies were concentrated on their staffroom campaign. It
was also clear that the well-meaning but self-conscious treatment of
black pupils in their classroom did not satisfy the immediate needs of
the black students. The multi-racial input of the 'Crusaders' into
classroom work did not appear to have much effect on the black
pupils in the lesson, though, it must be said, it did make these lessons
and teachers more popular and liked. These teachers were regarded
as more caring, less strict and more approachable.[8] For example,
though one young black woman described Rachel as 'sweet', this did
not mean that these teachers had the trust or confidence of the young
black women in their classes. The young black women explained
that they often felt patronised and were aware of these teachers'
efforts to be 'nice'. 'You think he is nice and all. He'll come up and
speak to you nice, but you can't trust him, he'll stab you in the back'
(Verne: black girl, fifth year, St Hilda's, talking about Mr Sutton, the
fifth year head).

The black girls stated clearly that they did not feel the classes of
certain 'Crusader'-type teachers to be the best, although they were
the most pleasant to be in. The girls frequently articulated their

desire for more structured lessons. For example, Mr Mahon's relaxed approach to his English lessons, in which he invited fifth years to contribute by recounting their own experiences, was met by bemused non-participation by the young black women in the class. These girls, who sat throughout the lesson in the back of the classroom, looked on while others carried on doing 'prep'. One girl said what she thought of the lesson: 'I never can understand what he is on about. What he want to know all that for?' [sic]

Other pupils found their teachers' efforts to include in the lesson what they considered to be socially relevant 'black' experiences amusing, as Brenda explained: 'Miss, it was a laugh, Miss Spencer made Verne be a social worker, right, and then I was sent to her as I was caught missing school, right. . . . It was funny, miss' (Anita, talking about her fifth-year drama lesson). Not only did the girls in this group have no experience of truanting, they had never been near a social worker. Ms Spencer had assumed that such experiences were a reality for the pupils in her class, an unwarranted assumption.

Ms Spencer's perspective on the lesson was markedly different from that articulated by the black girls in the class, as she explained: 'It was a very good session, the black kids got into it. It's important that the material is socially relevant for them. I think they could really understand what it was all about, it was good.'

In conclusion, the evidence suggests that the outcome of the 'Crusader' anti-racist campaign was less productive than they themselves believed. The efforts of these well-intentioned teachers were lost on both their colleagues and their pupils: the former alienated, and the latter they neglected, if not misunderstood. This failure of the anti-racist campaign was not only attributable to the way they went about things and the attitude of their colleagues, but was also the inevitable outcome of the fundamental flaws in their philosophy (Gilroy 1990).

4 The 'Liberal Chauvinists'

Unlike the 'Crusaders' the 'Liberal Chauvinists' were not campaigners for social justice. These teachers did, however, attempt to 'understand' (albeit only within the context of their own perspective), the cultural, class and gender characteristics of the various minorities they came into contact with. Armed with information, mostly gleaned from secondary sources such as television, books, travels, friends, rather than personal experience, these liberally inclined teachers were often convinced, with a curious arrogance that characterised the 'Liberal Chauvinists', that when it came to their students, they knew best. There were many examples of such liberally orientated staff in the schools in the study. Approximately 25 per cent of the teachers held beliefs that would classify them in this category.

There were many different types of 'Liberal Chauvinism' to be found among the staff in both the schools, each form having its own unique characteristics and therefore specific outcome for the young black women who found themselves on the receiving end of this type of 'unintentional' racism. Turning to an examination of one of these forms of 'Liberal Chauvinism', I cite first the case of Mr Sutton.

Sutton, the fifth year head at St Hilda's, believed that he, better than any other member of staff, 'understood' *his* black female students. In his efforts to 'understand' the young black women in his classrooms, Mr Sutton had become preoccupied with the issue of the sexuality of the black female pupils in the fifth year, as indeed were many other members of staff. It seemed that for Mr Sutton the answer to everything, when it came to young black women – success, failure; good or bad behaviour, happiness or sadness – lay in an explanation that had as its central causal concern the dynamic of black female sexuality. In the fifth year at St Hilda's there were several Band 1 black girls who were not achieving as expected, he explained:

> I do feel ethnic monitoring or at least keeping a record of black pupils could help us understand what's going on better. It has occurred to me, just by looking at the reports, that something is very wrong, very wrong indeed: how much is actually concerned with behaviour and not achievement? In a few weeks these girls suddenly do badly . . . so much going on inside them. What I mean is that they are maturing, becoming young ladies. It seems at this point their performance slips . . . as if school is, well beneath them. Yes, I do think many of them begin to feel that school is beneath them.

The fifth-year reports of the black female pupils, written by Sutton and other members of staff, reaffirmed the popular notion linking sexual maturity to levels of achievement. In these reports, which make often overtly sexist comments regarding particular feminine characteristics, behaviour is employed as the medium through which achievement and maturity are assessed. The following extracts from the school reports of young black women in the fifth year illustrate my point:

Sandra must learn to behave like a woman if she is to be treated like one. . . .
(Mr Farr: fifth-year class tutor commenting on Sandra, aged 16)

Very able and mature girl capable of doing well in future years. Her attitude to work and manner and punctuality are all worthy of mention. Well done!
(Mr Sutton: fifth year head commenting on Verne, aged 16)

Charm and good manners are as commendable in a young woman as work and punctuality!
(Mr Sutton: commenting on Donna, aged 16)

It is clear from this report that the staff and I feel that Frances is maturing gradually. I hope the sensible approach has not come too late.
(Mr Sutton: commenting on Frances, aged 16)

Sandra is a good girl who has to work hard to do well. She has responded well recently to appeals for mature behaviour. With the world of work looming on the horizon, and a change in behaviour she is capable of passing a number of subjects in the exams.
(Mr Sutton: commenting on Sandra, aged 16)

It was not uncommon to find members of staff in both schools complaining, generally, of the 'naïve and immature' approach all fifth-year students had towards their exams and to their future. As one teacher explained: 'They simply do not take them [exams] seriously. They have no idea of what is required of them in the real world' (Mr Gavin: Mathematics teacher, St Hilda's).

However, when discussing black girls the teachers would also complain more specifically about boyfriends, aggressive and unruly behaviour, and in general, assertiveness, which was often interpreted as being 'cocky'. It appeared that the girls' status as young women had contradictory outcomes in the way they were regarded. Being mature, on the one hand, was seen as the explanation for responsibility and taking schoolwork seriously. On the other hand, a 'developed' sense of maturity was regarded as a reason for lack of concentration and dissatisfaction with schooling. In this regard the black girls could not win. Their sexuality was perceived to be continually at odds with their educational achievement. Whether 'developed' or not, it was clear that their sexuality had to be contained.

This need to move towards a containment of black female sexuality was never more apparent than in the case of Anita, the young black fifth-former who became pregnant just before she was to take her final exams. The reaction to Anita's pregnancy revealed that the control of black female sexuality presented a constant and underlying concern with regard to the schooling of young black women. The 'scandal' of Anita's pregnancy became known when her father rang the school to say that she would no longer be attending. Mr Sutton was as intrigued as he was excited at being in on the 'scandal'. He explained in hushed tones:

> Anita has disgraced herself . . . . I had a suspicion when she begun to miss so much school, it wasn't like her. Don't tell any of the others, keep it between us, if they know, well, other parents, the school . . . what a waste, honestly these girls will get themselves into such situations. Anita was such a lovely girl.

The shame of the event was evident.[9] Mr Gavin, who was also a form tutor for the fifth year, had this to say of the incident: 'What a pity. . . . I was very disappointed in Anita.'

The outcome of the situation was that the staff who had previously professed a interest in Anita's academic ability as one of the most promising students of the fifth year washed their hands of the matter. They made no attempt to assist her in her studies or to advise her on her educational future. The issue was not to be discussed and Anita was warned not to come to school in her 'state'. Because the obvious expression of her sexuality had caused the school embarrassment, Anita was now regarded as being an immoral individual, and as such a bad influence on her peers.[10] The perceived 'understanding' by the 'Liberal Chauvinists' towards their black female pupils was short-lived when Anita's situation was judged from their own moral (and cultural) standpoint.

However, the theory pertaining to black female sexuality was only one of a number of 'informed' beliefs held by the 'Liberal Chauvinists' to explain the educational performance of the black girls in their classrooms. Ideas about the nature of the cultural and family background of West Indian female pupils were also culturally 'distanced' and as such often misunderstood. For example, it was not uncommon to find that many teachers felt that their black pupils possessed a cultural handicap that inhibited their successful educational participation. This belief, it must be stressed, emanated from a so-called 'informed' perspective that these teachers thought they had about West Indian life, and was therefore different in kind from the attitude displayed by the 'Overt Racists', who held a similar but more genetically orientated view.

In staffroom discussions teachers, who regarded themselves as informed, often showed a complete lack of understanding when it came to the cultural values or social lives of young black people. There was often surprise (and horror) at the extent to which young black girls helped and were expected to help with household chores. Some 'progressive' members of staff, most of whom were women themselves, felt it was a handicap to the girls' educational advancement. In one instance a mother, who was herself an educational welfare officer, was summoned to the school to be told to stop 'putting upon her daughter'. Ms Parker, believing in her estimation and using the yardstick of her own experience, that this was indeed not only an endemic but also detrimental aspect of West Indian culture, decided that this was an explanation for Sherry's recent deterioration in her (high-ability) work. She took matters into her own hands, saying:

> She [Sherry's mother] is one of those that believes you must work hard to get anywhere, you know, to work and work to better one's self. I think she's too hard on Sherry. She drives herself so hard, she's now started fainting during school time. It is emotional stress if you ask me. I understand the father left home, then came back and he treats them very badly, they have no beds at the moment, and if Sherry does not help at home she gets no food. A bit of a problem, don't you think? It is difficult to know what to do. We are considering sending her to the school psychologist'.

Whatever the cause of Sherry's distress over her schoolwork, the pathological sensationalism of Ms Parker's explanation displayed in this extract had clearly been fed by the impoverished images she had of cruel black men and over-ambitious black women. Yet Ms Parker had derived her explanation from her own evaluation of West Indian culture.

It was apparent that pictures of black pupils coming from, on the whole, socially deprived backgrounds, and thus in need of care and assistance, were being pieced together from information teachers read or saw and understood within their own cultural framework. These assessments of their pupils had important consequences for the black girls in their care. Their ideas impinged on the expectations and attitudes they had toward certain girls, who became labelled as problem children or not from the impressions that they derived, from often very limited contact with the parents of the girls.

Lisa and Deborah both had parents who came regularly to the PTA at St Theresa's to help out. These girls came from what were considered to be middle-class, professional, black families (that is, the father had the professional job and not the mother), and were regarded by Ms Parker as 'lovely young ladies'. In contrast to Sherry's mother, she described Lisa's mother as 'Well dressed and attractive, keen, and worth meeting'.

On the other hand, Miriam was seen as deviant, not least because of her parents:

> Miriam is not reliable. . . . Her mother, well, she is nice, but so disorganised. If you ring they never know where their daughters are or what they are up to . . . still in bed sometimes and they have to boot them out. I understand they never pay their bills, electricity is turned off, no bath etc.

Here social problems were turned into character deficiencies, whereas in the next example Mr Scott claimed a black mother who had principles had, in effect, 'personality problems': 'She thinks all books are "racist". I hear she's crazy anyway, tears the books up and throws them away. She's one of those real "hardliners". I think her behaviour is affecting her daughter.'

If, on the other hand, black parents were less assertive, for whatever reason, it was interpreted as a measure of their cultural and educational 'backwardness'. Mr Gavin, for example, had this to say of the parents of a West Indian pupil who was in 'trouble' with the school: 'they are very decent people, but they never come to school. They are a bit overawed by the whole thing.'

The issue of black parental 'fear' of the educational system was often brought up in staff meetings to account for the poor parental participation in all aspects of schooling. In contrast, the matter of the school failing in its role to encourage parental attendance was not emphasised. It would seem that the black parents could not win: they were equally a 'problem' whether they spoke out or remained silent.

Unrealistic expectations and over-ambition was another aspect of West Indian 'culture' with which the 'Liberal Chauvinists' preoccupied themselves. It was felt among the staff that these demands were imposed on the children of West Indian households as a matter of course. The staff tended to regard the hopes of parents for their children not as considered aspirations, but as symptomatic of what they 'knew' to be the unrealistic cultural orientation of black families (an over-ambition that also determined what they considered to be the unacceptable levels of discipline in West Indian households). Thus the common complaint of 'too high aspirations' among West Indian parents was met with a general concern among the 'Liberal Chauvinists' that the daughters of such unreasonable parents should be preserved from such demands, as the following example shows.

Linda's mother is very strict, one of those religious West Indian families, you know. She even says 'God bless you' when you ring. Now, she wants Linda to do 'A' Level RE, but she hasn't got a clue about her daughter. She's not even up to grade 3 CSE. She lives in another world, both of them.

(Ms Parker: fifth-year head at St Theresa's, discussing Linda, aged 16)

Ms Wallace, Careers mistress, counsellor and English teacher at St Theresa's, felt deeply committed to 'her girls'. She was indeed a dedicated teacher with a long-standing reputation for 'caring and helping', yet she too harboured her convictions about the 'hopeless' position concerning the future of most of the black girls with whose charge she was entrusted.[11] She was prepared to discuss her concerns about individual fifth-year girls:

Miriam is being unrealistic. . . . She is not equipped academically or as a person to do probation work or any sort of social work, she will only be disappointed, yet another case of one who wants to be but won't be. But how do you deal with these situations, you tell me, it is very touchy.

(Four years later, in a follow-up study, Miriam had completed the social studies course she had wanted to do at the local FE college in Brixton)

Laurie I would call a fairly competent sort of girl, but she needs to focus more clearly on what she really will be able to do.

(Laurie was an outstanding tennis player with high hopes of becoming professional, but this was considered unrealistic by the school. She also had excellent academic credentials.)

Of Rubina, who wanted to study law and showed every indication that she was capable academically of pursuing such a career (she already had several CSE and 'O' level passes from her previous year in the fifth form), Ms Wallace was not prepared to offer any undue encouragement. She said: 'She may go on to do 'A' Levels, but she is so ambitious, may be a bit too anxious.'

Ms Wallace's pessimistic assessment of these high ability and achievement-orientated young black women was not shared by the black careers officer, Ms Forte, who visited St Theresa's on a regular basis to interview the girls and counsel them on their future choices. Ms Forte had views of her own, contrary to Ms Wallace, concerning the girls' capabilities: 'I think Miriam is fully capable of undertaking a social work course. . . . Ms Wallace presumes sometimes that these girls have less of a mind than they really do.'

Ms Wallace, however, remained adamant about the way in which she saw things. In a meeting she confidently explained to Ms Forte and myself the cause of black disadvantage:

> We have our fair share of deprived girls here. You know who they are: they miss work, always absent, truant, come late, sometimes it's quite appalling. Then they turn around and say to you, 'Can't do it . . . will you help us?' How can you if they do not help themselves? They feel once you are here you have to think for them. They just have to learn to do it for themselves. They are on the verge of entering the world of work, the real world we are told, and they have not a thought in their head about anything let alone a career.

Opinions such as these were clear obstacles to the girls' educational progress. Ms Wallace's attitude set up in the classroom a situation of cause and effect. The astute girls in her class often minimised their efforts and involvement in her lessons, and in doing so increased the amount of attention she as a teacher felt necessary to give them. However, this was only one way in which such negative teaching attitudes affected the girls. It was far more common to witness more obvious and direct negative assessments, as the following example demonstrates.

Ms Andrews, a third-year mistress, explained that one of her third-year students, a black girl, was insistent on taking History as an examination subject for the future. However, she felt:

Andrea is just not capable and she has been strongly advised not to. She is disorganised and a lazy girl, and slow. Even if she were able to do the CSE she could not complete the course work. She wants to do it so badly but we know she'll fail. I cannot allow it.

Such concern could easily be regarded as an honest assessment, advice that, in order to avoid disappointment, sensibly takes into account the limitations of a pupil's ability. However, when another teacher's evaluation of Andrea is taken into consideration, this assessment begins to seem unfair. Another teacher revealed: 'It is not that she [Andrea] is lazy or not able to manage, it is just that she tries too hard. For instance she'll rewrite four lines in one lesson just to get it right and looking good.'

Tomlinson (1981b:59) has found that many teachers do operate within a framework of stereotypes which are more often reinforced than negated by pupil response. She argues that it was not uncommon to find that teachers regarded their West Indian pupils as generally slow, docile and underachievers on the one hand, and hyperactive and anti-authoritarian on the other. In the case of Andrea the primary response of the teacher was to categorise her as slow and lazy. This meant that the teacher overlooked and failed to encourage the qualities of perseverance and commitment that Andrea obviously had. Thus, rather than attempting to develop her potential, Ms Andrews labelled Andrea as lazy and slow, relegating her to the category of 'difficult and problematic'.

Sharon, a bright fifth-year pupil at St Theresa's, found herself in a similar situation to Andrea, although unlike Andrea she had been classified as over-ambitious rather than slow. Ms Parker, her form mistress, explained:

She is aiming far too high. I think it is fair to say that all the staff are concerned, she will only be disappointed in September. But we feel she is only capable of 5–6 CSEs. There were tears all round when we discussed [with her mother] that she will have to really drop one subject.

Ms Parker's rationale for giving Sharon this advice was obvious. She explained that her family circumstances were such that overloading Sharon with work was wrong:

Her mother works nights, she's a nurse I believe. There are many social problems in the family. I think the father left and there are

small children involved. Sharon has to help out and we just don't
think she can cope.

Sharon desperately wanted to do all the subjects she was trying for as
they were necessary for her to gain access to the social work course
she wanted to enrol in for the following year. Parker, however, in
the girl's 'best interests' felt that the course should not be her primary
consideration, and rather than offer any support or understanding,
strongly advised Sharon to give up what was to her a very important
course.[12]

This statement of Mr Sutton's reveals the paternalism that charac-
terises a 'Liberal Chauvinistic' approach: 'I get on well with her
[Gina], *you have to understand her,* if she feels someone is against her
she reacts in a violent way.'[13]

In conclusion, there were numerous examples of teachers' negative assessments, most of which were based on what they believed to
be 'informed judgement'. These negative assessments often led to the
curtailment of opportunities that should have been available to the
black girls in the study in view of their ability and attainment.

5 The 'Black Teacher'

There is an expectation that, with a positive policy of recruitment
towards black teachers, not only will it present a more representative
picture of the population of the inner city, but that they will also be
placed in the forefront of the demand for a more progressive and
egalitarian educational system. However, in the schools studied the
black members of staff, who numbered only four, did not participate
in the obvious arena that had been constructed to encourage such
change. The anti-racist campaign, which on the whole was monopo-
lised by the 'Crusaders', did not attract black support, as Mr Green,
a young black male teacher at St Hilda's, explained: 'I just let them
get on with their business. I don't bother with them. They feel they
know what it is all about so who am I to say. I find it just gets on my
nerves, I keep well out of it.' [*sic*]

This negative feeling about the 'liberal white tokenism' that
dominated the race issue in schools was articulated by the other black
teachers:

The ILEA has set about 'investigating' the 'problem of race'.
Everyone is rushing around 'investigating race', talking about

'running out of time', having to do it now. A curious way to go about things.

(Ms Lewis: head of Biology department, St Theresa's)

It was not that these black members of staff did not sympathise with the need to reassess the issue of race in the schools, but that they shared[14] a definite and alternative perspective on the nature of the black educational dilemma and the solution to that problem. This orientation was clear from the statements these teachers made about the role and development of multi-racial education. For example, when Ms Lewis was asked what she felt about multi-racial education and equal opportunities policies, she said: 'So what about them? What needs to change, if you ask me, is ourselves and our attitudes as teachers, rather than the girls.'

As a Science teacher in an all-girls school, Ms Lewis had particular views concerning the issue of equal opportunities and Science teaching for all the girls, whether black or white:

More important than multi-racial education is the way certain subjects are taught to all pupils regardless. The way science is taught should be looked at. It is often the way science is approached that prevents girls from seeing it as useful or enjoying it . . . nothing is that difficult if it is taught properly. Why should physics or chemistry be defined as difficult or more challenging than other subjects? All subjects require different skills and approaches, if it clicks, if it is enjoyable, and if you have got the knack, then why should it be difficult?

In this school, like everywhere, they say and encourage only 'clever' girls to do chemistry and physics 'O' level. Why should science be reserved for the 'clever' girls? Why should you be 'clever' to understand maths? . . . It is just our own values about cleverness linked to science. Now equal opportunities are recommending as a positive policy that 'clever', more able girls do physics and chemistry at 'O' level and then go on straight to do 'A' level biology. This is their way of trying to make more girls take part and do more science, but it does not get to the heart of the problem.

The opinion that black pupils should maximise their learning capacity during traditional and structured classroom contact hours was also a common theme among black members of staff. For example, Dr Ashraf, an Asian Science teacher at St Hilda's, had this to say about mother-tongue teaching:

There is a lot of emphasis on Spanish and Italian languages here, being Catholic many come from those parts. It's a waste. Asian languages in school is wasting the children's time when they could be learning other things to get them a job. It should be done at home, we don't need the school to tell us who we are or what to speak. Time in school should be spent on learning.

As the issue of role models is often discussed in relation to the recruitment of black teachers, an aspect that is worth investigating is pupil response to their presence. It was apparent in the schools that the race of the teacher was not as significant as the quality of their teaching and their ability to communicate with the girls. Of course the race of the teacher did automatically increase their ability to empathise with the girls and so increased their popularity, as the girls explained:

Ms Lewis, she's a good teacher. She makes you work, but she's always fair.

(Fifth-year black girl)

She never picks on anyone, not like Ms Webster . . . best of all she never shouts at you.

(Fifth-year black girl commenting on Ms Lewis)

The feeling was mutual: the exchange between black teacher and black pupil showed no elements of favouritism or special recognition; they were regarded simply as pupils by the teachers and teachers by the pupils.[15] Mr Green demonstrated this when he warned me about several black male students in the school: 'Those boys, they are trouble makers. They try to disrupt everything for you. Just ignore them and keep out of their way, that is what we all do.'

Similarly, Ms Lewis explained that she did not give any particular preference to the young black women she taught just because she herself was a black woman. She explained her philosophy on the matter, a philosophy that was in marked contrast to that expressed by many of her white colleagues and documented earlier in this chapter.

No matter who we are we can only do what we can . . . there is no point in trying to be or do what you can't. No matter if you are black or white we all have limitations. The important thing is to recognise what those limitations are in terms of your academic ability and work on your strong points.

Being a black woman and having a black perspective on issues concerning the pupils was, as in the case of Ms Forte, the careers liaison officer at St Theresa's, of immense value when it came to advising and understanding the girls' needs. In her realistic appraisal of the career situation for young black women she was able to relate the desire for certain jobs to family background, the migrant experience and social class influences among West Indians. As a black female careers officer, Ms Forte felt she was in a difficult position, but she did not give the girls false hope or misleading information just because she felt that black women should aspire as high as they could, she explained:

> As a careers officer my role is to prepare them for a job. To broaden their interests and to provide information, but also to be aware of how we as careers officers can affect their opportunities. . . . It is difficult to assess what job they would like and how to give advice. You can't say, 'no, you can't be such and such.' You have to be realistic, it just may not be possible. Ultimately, it's your job to help them stop wasting time wanting to be a doctor by giving them realistic advice. Some girls, for example, are late developers. You have to then just give them the facts and help them make their mind up. If they want to work hard give them the time and don't say you can't. They may feel you are discouraging them if you don't give them alternative advice, but then as a black officer, and this goes for black teachers, we are perceived as part of the system, the authority. It is very frustrating.

Another distinctive feature of the black teachers in the study was that they were all involved in further study of one sort or another in an effort to enhance their own career prospects. Mr Green, the Social Science teacher at St Hilda's, left the school during my time spent there doing fieldwork. He moved to a larger, more 'progressive' comprehensive school. His immediate aim was job satisfaction, though he also had his eye on the future by studying for a part-time MA in education. Likewise, Ms Forte sought to forward her career, even though she was a trained social worker; she had been also studying for a part-time MA (at the University of London, Goldsmiths' College), which she had just finished. She described her reasons for continuing her studies:

> I've been going to evening class for the past five years. It was so difficult sometimes but I can say now 'I've done it'. I am proud,

but it was a sacrifice. It was worth it. I came to England when I was 13 and it has always been a struggle, I've always had to work hard. But this degree now means that I can move on . . . this job is just not stretching enough and now I want to try something else. [sic]

Ms Lewis too was highly motivated. She had achieved the status as head of department in her school and was much respected as a competent teacher and colleague. Like the black girls they were teaching, these black teachers were resourceful in building up their careers by whatever means available.

On the whole, everyday working relationships between the black members of staff and their white colleagues were amiable. However, in one instance racial strife in the classroom caused one black teacher to complain about the lack of support and understanding among white colleagues. Dr Ashraf, a Chemistry teacher at St Hilda's, had been having a great deal of trouble with one particular fifth-year Chemistry group. The racism of the pupils was evident as he became the object of their abuse. The class constantly made fun of him, mimicking his 'Indianness' and calling him derogatory Indian names. The pupils even began to boycott his lessons and taunt him that they were not going to attend the final exam. These events caused Dr Ashraf much distress. He had appealed to the headmaster, Mr Madden, and the staff, but found not only disbelief but little sympathy and support. They, he felt, regarded him as an incompetent teacher and was aware that the non-entry of substantial numbers of fifth-formers for the Chemistry examination would fuel that belief. However, though Dr Ashraf had outstanding credentials[16] and was a dedicated teacher, he was aware of the lack of recognition and racism he had suffered not only in the job market, but also from his colleagues, who judged him primarily on his accent and ability to speak English. The lack of support over the fifth-form incident, he felt, was a further insult to his integrity. He was aware that in the staffroom he was regarded as very much an outsider:

I feel very alone. I can't tell anyone anything. I am aware that a lot of what is going on is because I'm Indian and everyone else here is Catholic. Parents, teachers, together they will say I'm not able to manage the class. Parents, they especially have a lot to do with it. They influence their children at home and that is why they feel they can come here and say and do these things like this.

The irony of this incident was that it took place in a school, St Hilda's, in which the staff were most vociferous that racism was not present among them.

In conclusion, the experiences and values of the black teachers in the study differed radically from those of the white teachers. On the whole, the black teachers were more in tune with the needs of their black female pupils, often offering a more positive solution to the education of the black child.

CONCLUSION: THE STRATEGIC AVOIDANCE OF RACISM

The evidence of this study shows that while young black women (who clearly displayed their positive self-esteem), challenged their teachers' expectations of them (expectations that were often characterised by overt racism on the one hand or unintentional racism on the other), they were in no position in the 'power hierarchy' to counteract any negative outcomes of these interpretations.

All too often the recognition of these negative assessments led the girls to look for alternative strategies with which to 'get by'. These strategies, such as not taking up a specific subject or not asking for help, were employed by the girls as the only means of challenging their teachers' expectations of them, and as such were ultimately detrimental to the education of the pupils concerned.

However, the attitudes and orientations of black teachers presented a positive example of how some of the processes of disadvantage could be avoided. These teachers neither patronised nor misinterpreted their black students' reactions and were insistent on the maintenance of high standards of teaching and learning.

Chapter 5

Entering the world of work

It is widely reported that young black people, both male and female, are more likely to use the services of the official recruitment agencies when seeking employment in comparison to their white peers.[1] For young blacks, occupational placement is least likely to be the outcome of social networks, family relationships and other informal channels. The occupational location of the parental generation of these youths, the migrant generation, can be seen to contribute to the weaknesses of such internal self-perpetuating recruitment practices.

In the 1950s West Indians found work in what in the 1980s and 1990s have become declining and restricted areas of the economy. Occupying such a disadvantaged location in the economy reduces the opportunity of working-class West Indians to reproduce their labour-market networks. Furthermore, the prevalence of racism in tandem with the hierarchical nature of work-place structures affects the influence most West Indians have on recruitment practice. The reliance on formal and official information that this engenders makes young black people particularly vulnerable to the quality and type of information they receive. Young black women depend on such sources to gain vital access to information on two counts: firstly, to find out about new occupational and career possibilities, jobs previously not accessible to an earlier generation: and secondly, to secure recruitment to a specific job.

In order to address these issues I investigate the nature of and access to occupational information and advice available to the young black women in the study. Such an analysis requires an examination of the role of the school in its ultimate function, that of occupational placement. Thus I look at the way in which the various services and agencies that are involved in the process of occupational placement for the school leaver operate.

The Careers Service and agencies like the MSC are investigated. I also examine the provisions within the schools. Careers lessons, courses that focus on vocational preparation, such as Personal and Social Education programmes, and YTS-orientated schemes, are given detailed consideration. I also investigate the type of advice and information received by students while they make crucial choices in their school career during their third, fifth and sixth years.

THE CAREERS EDUCATION PROGRAMME

One official information resource available to young black women in school was the Careers Education Programme (CEP). Both of the schools in the study complied with the now formalised but nevertheless minimal recommendations set out in a report undertaken by HMI in 1973 (DES 1973). This report, apart from an increased concern in preparing the school leaver for the transition to work, showed no ideological shift from the previous 1948 and 1965 statements on the role of careers advice. The core of the career guidance philosophy remained 'a clear understanding of self in the important task of making the appropriate personal decision' (Schools Council 1972:38).

Thus the 1973 brief emphasised the development of school leaver/pupil self-awareness, occupational awareness and decision making. Tasks such as letter writing, personal appearance, interview techniques and acceptable employee behaviour formed the focus of the CEP. For example, St Theresa's, in a report outlining the main aims of their Careers department, state that the goals of their programme were:

(1) To develop self-awareness, appreciation of their own strengths and weaknesses and tactics for improvement.
(2) To enable pupils to make realistic decisions about choices within the curriculum.
(3) To develop an awareness of the world of work – its restrictions, responsibilities and challenge.

It was apparent that in the programme the labour market was assumed to be static, occupational location being determined largely as a consequence of individual choice (within, of course, the context of personal constraint). In the face of rising unemployment and the reproduction of racial and sexual divisions at work the philosophy of the CEP is clearly in question (Ainley 1988).

Caught up in the contradictions of a careers programme, which suggests on the one hand that advice should be based on individual choice, and placed within institutions that, on the other hand, 'have few pretensions toward an academic education' (Tomlinson 1987: 98), are well-meaning teachers and careers officers.

Both St Hilda's and St Theresa's offered a poorly resourced and ineffectual service. The schools did comply with HMI minimal requirements to provide career guidance in the 13+ curriculum. However, because provision remained only in the form of recommendations with guidelines, standards of the CEP varied greatly in quality and quantity between each school (VanDyke 1985).

A universal feature of the CEP was, however, its status on the periphery of the school curriculum. The head of Careers at St Theresa's complained that there was no adequate time-table allowance for careers advice sessions. A minimum of one lesson a week was not feasible for most of the fifth year because of lack of time and a reluctance to withdraw them from 'examinable' subject lessons. The outcome of which was that two-thirds of fifth-formers had one Careers lesson every other week and one-third had none. The third and the fourth years had scheduled some sort of careers input into their curriculum every other week, but only as part of the 'Living Programme'; a general course focusing on personal and social education, covering subjects such as health, sex education and environmental issues.

However, during the year I spent at St Theresa's the 'Living Programme' was withdrawn from the lower school curriculum because of what was defined as 'discipline problems', but what appeared in reality to be inadequate supervision and tutoring. There were no qualified teachers to take these classes; teachers with a free time-table slot were allocated to these secondary-status teaching quotas.

The sixth year had no careers guidance lessons. As the sixth-form prospectus explained, 'Careers are left up to the pupils' own motivation.' Meetings could, however, be arranged with a very busy and elderly sixth-form mistress who was also head of Careers for the sixth as well as a Chemistry teacher, and whose main function was to help with the filling in of UCCA forms or college applications.

At St Hilda's the provision for CEP was equally poor. One fifth-year class had no classroom available in which the lesson could take place so the year had to sit in the library for 'quiet reading and prep'. The sixth years, like those at St Theresa's, had no time-table allowance allocated for careers advice, nor were they given much support or encouragement. On Wednesday afternoons during their General Studies programme they were advised to 'seek assistance'. They were told in their sixth-form prospectus: 'It is up to you to make the Careers Service and advice work for you by using them efficiently, and by asking for advice and guidance.'

As the provision for resources for the CEP was never statutorily laid down by the DES, it was left to the individual school to allocate what it deemed adequate. In both schools in the study the personal enthusiasm and ingenuity of the Careers tutor determined what could be provided. The 'Careers rooms' in St Hilda's and St Theresa's were kept locked. They were also both located in inaccessible and unattractive parts of the school. At St Theresa's it was a small dark room situated behind the stage in the assembly hall. At St Hilda's it was in the most isolated wing of the top floor of a teaching block (fourth floor), near the toilets.

The budget allocation was also very small. In St Theresa's the allowance for the academic year 1982–1983 for the entire school was just £400, an increase of £150 since 1978. As a consequence, the Careers departments in both schools were ill equipped. Old books, containing outdated concepts about work and the types of jobs available, were often torn and incomplete but were still being displayed unattractively on shelves in the Careers room. Particularly notable was the limited range of professions available to girls and the prevalence of dated, gender-stereotyped literature.

In accordance with the DES requirements the schools had teachers designated with career responsibilities. In both cases the English and Social Studies teachers were appointed Careers tutors. In this capacity they employed their own experience (believed to be more appropriate because of their interest in the humanities), rather than any formal training in the field of counselling. However, the responsibilities of 'doubling up' their commitments as a teacher with their role as an adviser were not satisfactory, as Ms Wallace, the Careers mistress and English and Social Studies teacher at St Theresa's explained: 'A heavy teaching time-table of 25 out of 30 periods and so many added responsibilities is not conducive to inspired thought, action or time to co-operate with colleagues over the careers of girls.' This sentiment was echoed by Ms Reed the English, Social Studies and Careers mistress at St Hilda's at the beginning of the new school year when she considered the prospect of a new fifth year: 'Oh God, yet another set to get through. Just finished one lot and now another to go. . . . It's a demanding time ahead, a heavy load.'

For the pupils the message concerning careers was clear. It was not to be taken seriously. Regarded as free time on the time-table, Careers lessons were used as 'prep' or homework time, often to the exasperation of the assigned teacher who had the unenviable task of teaching this ill-defined and woolly area of the curriculum. In these lessons the pupils were set unimaginative tasks such as filling in dummy application forms or answering questionnaires. Role-play, where one pupil interviews another, was seen as a chance for amusement by the participants and often degenerated into chaos. One fifth-year girl described these unstructured and poorly planned sessions as 'a real waste of a period'. In general the pupils would either do the required task as quickly as they could, and then proceed to get on with lesson 'prep' or homework, or just sit or gossip while the teacher managed to get some of her own preparation done.

Descriptions of the Careers classes I observed are revealing. Among the pupils in both schools, three responses to Careers lessons were identifiable. These three responses corresponded to the ability level of the pupils concerned and were easily observable because of the system of streaming by ability that both schools engaged in.

The first response was that of the Band 3 pupils. These pupils, designated as being of low ability, saw Careers as a free lesson. In St Theresa's the classes were made up mainly of black girls. The lesson would be extremely noisy and chaotic (though those who chose to do their 'prep' sat undisturbed in the back of the room). During one session several girls danced to a Michael Jackson tape to pass the time after completing the set work. At St Hilda's it was much the same, though the lessons here were co-educational with both black and white pupils. The general strategy employed by these pupils was to make a boring lesson entertaining. They would 'muck about', tease one another, throw books, ask for unnecessary help, and fight. To these pupils Careers sessions were a total waste of time; when asked, few had any real idea of what they would really like to do – the question being redundant, as most of these pupils were designated for YTS and knew that to be their fate. However, it must be said that the black girls, in contrast to their white peers, had a clearer idea of what they would like to do and showed a keen interest in finding out more about what they could possibly do.

The second response was that of the black pupils of average to high ability. In contrast to their peers, who had a predetermined future in the form of the YTS, these pupils were set apart by their desire for information. In response to the inadequate supply of career guidance they had so far received, these fifth-year pupils wanted to know from me about university and college courses, and various non-traditional female jobs and what they entailed. For example, in one class they were keen to know about careers in the law. They were also eager to learn about computing. It was clear from these sessions that these able girls had little idea about how to go about applying for jobs or the steps involved that would lead them down a chosen career path. In these sessions the girls were attentive and responsive. They expressed their interest in having sessions that provided information with which to enhance their own limited view of the job market, and the change this presented from their usual Careers class.

The third response was that of the girls of high ability. These girls were characterised by a degree of certainty about their future, though there was a distinction to be made here between the white and the black female pupils' attitudes. Several of the black girls of high ability fell into the category above, showing a strong need for good progressive guidance. However, in general these girls felt that they were fairly certain about what they were going to be doing in the future and therefore felt that careers advice was superfluous. In their lessons many girls finished off the set work and sat quietly doing 'prep'. However, on examination of their career choices both black and white girls who belonged to this group had chosen very traditional professional occupations and college courses. The black girls here were particularly prone to choosing 'gendered' careers orientated to social work. The lack of any imaginative careers guidance led many girls to reproduce safe and known career options.

In conclusion, the response of the girls to their Careers lessons was a clear indication of the poverty of their content and philosophy. The lessons were met with boredom and lack of interest and were clearly, as the pupils indicated, in their present form, 'a waste of time'. The need for good, positive and progressive advice was evident especially among the black girls, who, it is known, rely heavily on institutional channels for advice. In this study only 39 per cent of the young black women said they found their school CEP useful (in contrast to 70 per cent of their white peers). This clearly indicates the need for reform in this area of the school curriculum to assist these young women to make considered choices.

THE CAREERS SERVICE

The schools had the services of an external Careers officer provided by the local Careers Office, who interviewed pupils within school hours during their time at school. Each Careers officer was responsible for several schools in their district and worked by a system of pre-arranged interviews with an individual pupil at given times. When asked what they felt about these advice sessions, most girls resented having to take time out of normal lessons to go. However, in contrast to how they felt about CEP, 63 per cent of black girls said they found the service useful (compared to 30 per cent of white girls), indicating the importance that these girls placed on this source of information.

With the reliance that these girls placed on the Service, the sensitivity of the Careers officer to the needs of black female pupils is crucial. Ms Forte, a black Careers officer at St Theresa's, had a particular empathy with the black girls she advised, and was well liked. Her popularity was most likely the cause of the positive response given by many black girls to questions about the usefulness of careers advice in schools. However, in spite of her special insights into the black female experience, Ms Forte acknowledged the limitations of her role and her ability to change things. She was aware that the girls would not truly confide in her as she was seen as part of the authority structure.

On the whole the girls reported that the information they received was appropriate, especially when it came to deciding what college course to apply for and how to go about that application. However, the advice given was clearly built up on pre-existing career choices of the girls and did not encourage them to explore other labour-market possibilities. This inability of the Careers Service to foster innovation among young black women entering the labour market has had the effect of perpetuating, in the majority of cases, those career paths that were known to be feasible for black females in Britain. For example, many girls expressed their desire to do social work courses not because it was their ultimate ambition, but rather because it has been a traditionally acceptable, high-status career for black women, providing opportunities for advancing their education.

The function of the Careers Service is not only to provide the necessary information school leavers need for their decision-making process, but it is also involved in matching up pupils to compatible employers registered with them. In this capacity it has been suggested that the Careers Service plays a significant role in the reproduction of sexual and racial divisions in the labour market (Eggleston *et al*. 1986). It is argued that they act as 'gate- keepers' with regard to occupational placement and in particular the various YTS schemes (Austin 1984, 1987; Cross 1987a). In spite of this, the 1991 proposals to reform the careers service remain limited and conservative, focusing largely on organisational issues and the question of private-sector financing (*Guardian*, 30 April 1991).

However, in my study it was apparent that the careers officers who liaised with the schools were presented with pupils who had been already sorted according to their perceived levels of ability, initiative and performance. Records kept by the Careers mistress were based very much on her judgement concerning an individual pupil's characteristics. This, considered to be enabling background information, was given to the Careers officers to assist in their task of providing the appropriate advice. However, these reports were profoundly influenced by teacher assessments that, as we have seen with regard to black female pupils, were not always appropriate. Cicourel and Kitsuse (1977) note the impact that assessments, made about a pupil on the basis of their personal and social features, can have. They suggest that although in some cases information gained about a student through testing is important, in the majority of cases 'a student's occupational mobility may be more than incidentally contingent upon the sponsorship of organisational personnel who verify him to be a serious, personable, well-rounded student, with leadership potential' (p. 29).

The streaming and selection of pupils during five years of schooling meant that the Careers officers in their one or two visits with a pupil were presented with a child who had already been assessed whom they then had the task of placing in an appropriate job. This was clearly illustrated in St Theresa's YTS preparation programme. St Theresa's offered a course called 'Looking Forward' which, from as early as the fourth year, filtered out the low achievers from the rest of the school. This programme was part of a strategy aimed at structuring these girls' educational careers along what was considered to be 'a less demanding' path. By encouraging the uptake of less academic, but clearly vocational, options such as child development, combined with the nurturing of their acceptance that the only way to enter the job market was through the YTS, the school created the desire in girls for careers such as nursery nursing and typing. This left the Careers officers with the task of finding them a YTS placement that would suit them and their experience. Thus the placement of these black girls on inferior schemes[2] was not so much the Careers officer's responsibility, as it has been suggested. Furthermore, the role of the Careers officers in occupational placement could also be 'bypassed' by the recruitment drives of the 'managing agents': private employers who subscribed to the YTS. These managing agents, who could offer more desirable and higher-status jobs in private industry than other employers on the schemes, recruited directly from the schools themselves. As observed in the schools studied, these companies 'head-hunted' for mainly white recruits in schools that had a large percentage of white students.

CAREERS TALKS AND VISITS

Careers talks by invited speakers and organised visits to work establishments were another source of information made available to the girls to assist them in making their decisions about the future. Arranged by the Careers departments of the schools, some four to five such events could be expected in the fifth year. However, the content and quality of these talks and visits varied according to the orientation of the school and type of pupils to whom they were addressed. For example, St Theresa's had arranged talks to be given on subjects such as engineering ('Opening Windows on Engineering'), which were aimed at interesting the academically inclined. In contrast, St Hilda's, with its 'academic mediocrity' offered no such professionally orientated discussions. The talks at St Hilda's were directly related to the recruitment drives for trainees by various large private and public-sector employers; for example, Lloyds Bank, British Telecom and, for the second year running, Vidal Sassoon. St Theresa's, with its largely black and female-only intake, attracted less attention from such recruitment drives.

Lee and Wrench (1983) observe that it is common practice for some companies to recruit directly in this way, a process (as we have already noted) which can lead to indirect discrimination. They write: 'Some firms see liaison work as time well spent in disseminating knowledge about their firm . . . others see it as a ritual which has to be performed with no real payoff' (p. 40).

Reaction to these talks aimed at encouraging school leavers to join a specific firm or organisation varied according to the gender of the pupil. For example, it had a significant influence on the career choices of the white boys at St Hilda's. The numbers who stated that they wanted to be bank clerks or BT engineers was marked after the careers talks given by the the respective recruitment organisation. The talks affected the choices of those yet undecided. However, boys who wanted to do a specific City and Guilds course or apprenticeship remained unchanged after these talks.

There was no evidence that these talks influenced in any way the choices of the young black women in the study. This was partly to do with the orientation of the recruitment drives which were aimed at a male and white audience, but also because by the fifth year most black girls had a fairly sure idea of what they might like to be doing in the future. At whatever level, their plans on the whole, though not necessarily innovative, were well thought-out, and included a strategy for getting ahead.

The young black women were highly critical of the quality of the talks and the information they provided. This was illustrated in their objections to the Lloyds Bank talk at St Hilda's. Lloyds Bank had sent a middle-aged 'English gentleman' as their representative. For 20 minutes he proceeded to present an uninspired slide show illustrating the various types of jobs in banking. The slides showed an outdated range of jobs which he himself acknowledged in response to the pupils' queries about computers and word processors. The objections, however, came mainly from the girls, who felt that women were being represented at the lower levels of employment. The jobs for women were at the clerical level; tillers, secretaries and so on. The talk was clearly aimed not at City banking but at high street banking, as he explained encouragingly, 'You only need a few 'O' levels or a couple of good CSEs for paperwork.'

When the Lloyds representative said, 'You must be keen and polite', one black interjected, 'and white'. The slide show included no black people at all. After the talk the black girls picked up on this omission, as Verne said, 'No blacks, no women: it's sexist, it's racist; even if they'd have you, who wants to work there anyway!' The girls were clearly fed up and bored during the talk, as one girl explained, 'I could have been doing something useful, instead of wasting my time, I wanted to do my English homework.'

Many of these organised sessions were regarded as a waste of time by the staff involved but continued nonetheless. For example, the trip to Vidal Sassoon was seen as a chance to have an afternoon off by the fifth year. Though it was optional, and only a few white girls had any genuine interest in a career in hairdressing, that afternoon the whole of the fifth was deserted, much to the staff's relief, who took the opportunity to catch up on overdue work and go home early.

Like St Hilda's, St Theresa's had also organised several career visits. Their trips included visits to Scotland Yard, the London College of Fashion, King's College Hospital and the BBC. However, these visits during school time were only for the YTS-destined pupils on the 'Looking Forward' programme, pupils who, as one teacher explained, they were glad to get off their hands for the afternoon. As part of a work experience campaign for the other pupils, St Theresa's did offer a post-examination 'Community Service Programme' for one week. Here the girls did voluntary work in a hospital, school or nursery, an extension of the school's philanthropic tradition which, since the days of the grammar regime, the headteacher had highly valued.

Each of the schools in the study did have a tradition of inviting old pupils back to give talks about their work or study experiences. Using the 'old girls' network', St Theresa's would invite a past student who had succeeded in a professional career or attended university to talk to the sixth form once or twice a year. St Hilda's had a more novel way of introducing the world of work to prospective leavers. Here a group of students who had recently left organised a careers day for the fifth years, entitled 'Christian Employment'.

The day was put on by several students from the South London College Christian group. It was held in the rather depressing surroundings of the school hall and consisted of talks and sketches, interspersed at intervals throughout the day with discussions and workshops. Staff made an effort not to be present so as not to inhibit the 'atmosphere'. The theme of the day was clear: the perseverance of the individual. One organiser explained: 'There is no need to find yourself unemployed. It is up to you to get a job; it is up to you to try: the jobs are there. Call on God for help and guidance.'

The response to the day was varied. On the whole the Christian participants faced a hostile and cynical audience, particularly on the issue of unemployment (there was a lot of heckling and non-participation during the day). The black girls were clearly dissatisfied with the solutions they were being presented with and felt they had little in common with the speakers (all of whom were white). One black girl asked, 'You tell us what prospects of employment do we have on the dole.' Another remarked, 'So why bother with qualifications if there is no employment?' The answer came predictably from the panel: 'It is up to you to convince the employer to take you on.'

When asked what they got from the day, one young woman summed up the sentiments of the others when she said: 'Boring, man, waste a time. Who they trying to fool, ain't gonna be me, man, let me go home and stop wasting my time with these people.' [*sic*]

Lectures on the importance of the work ethic were clearly not what these girls wanted or needed. Another young black woman, in commenting on what she had derived from her day, expressed the need again for good, positive and structured advice and guidance. As she explained: 'In our discussion group we talked about going for an interview. That was the most helpful part of the whole day, the rest was a joke!'

FROM SCHOOL TO YTS: SELECTION AND RECRUITMENT

Both at St Theresa's and St Hilda's there was an active and systematic process of recruitment of pupils on to the YTS.[3] These recruitment drives were selective, and disproportionately affected pupils classified in the lower-ability ranges.

Lower-ability pupils at St Theresa's in particular were having their aspirations directed towards expecting a future with the YTS. In this school it was brought about by means of the 'Looking Forward' course: a programme that at the end of the fifth year actually placed them on a YTS scheme. The 'Looking Forward' course was presented as a programme for non-academic fifth-formers: 'to help them prepare for life after school in the form of preparation for work and leisure in a large city' (Quinquennial Review). It was described as a non-examination option (three periods a week) that began in the fifth year and for which the pupil was awarded an internal school certificate at the end. The course itself was ill-defined but sure of its aims. It was explained that there is no homework, no tests and only informal practical activity. The central part of the course consisted of: 'visits and outings . . . to practise the skills of public travelling and to learn more about work and leisure. It is important they can find their way. They have just been on a trip to Harrods' (Quinquennial Review).

The course was objectively a way of 'containing' difficult girls who missed their ordinary lessons by being sent off the school site for their practical activities. As one teacher explained wryly: 'It soon sorts them out. They don't want to be at school but after a bout of work experience they soon find out that they don't want to be at work either.'

The schools' attitude to YTS-destined pupils was clearly less than encouraging. They saw them as failures and disappointments relative to the successful academic pupils who were expected to seek their employment opportunities, through the traditional, *laissez-faire*, labour-market system. The course organiser, Ms Maxwell, expressed this discriminatory sentiment when she explained, 'If they're no good for college we send them on to YTS.'

Ms Forte, the Careers officer at St Theresa's, was, in view of Ms Maxwell's statement, justifiably concerned with the way the YTS was being used as a means of 'mopping up the unemployable'. She explained: 'I am worried about the YTS being used as an alternative to college courses. You can see it especially in areas such as catering.'

The YTS input into schools received low status; this was reflected in its time-tabling and budget priority. The 'Looking Forward' course had no resources, no rooms or materials. In the three years since it began this part of the curriculum had received no money.

Because the courses did not attempt to expand the girls' experiences or develop their prospects concerning what jobs could be available, the girls (the clear majority of whom were black), accepted and indeed aspired to their YTS fate. As Linda, a fifth-year Band 3 girl, explained:

> I want to go on to YTS doing training for a nursery nurse at the age group of 3–4 and 5-year-olds. I want to do this because while I am at home I take care of this age group [her sister's children] and have experience in feeding and changing them. I also did child development in school to help me.

Failing to inform or encourage them to take up any other type of work the course succeeded in reinforcing traditional ideas of what unskilled or semi-skilled women's work should be, such as shop work, clerical work or low-grade hospital work. Aspiring to 'care'-orientated careers such as nursery nursing precipitated their placement on to YTS schemes of a lower status (namely Mode B, now no longer in operation in that form) which could not guarantee any permanent employment opportunities (Austin 1984, 1987).[4]

St Hilda's had comparatively a much less structured approach to YTS recruitment than St Theresa's. Unlike St Theresa's, the curriculum did not contain a course directed to YTS-destined pupils; instead, the selection for the YTS was left up to 'free market forces' and the procedures of the Careers Service. The latter entailed self-referral to the Service or necessary agencies by the school leavers upon finding themselves in the job market and unemployed. The former implied the activities of private agencies, given a free hand at St Hilda's, who were involved in the business of the direct recruitment of school leavers.

The staff and headteacher at St Hilda's had a *laissez-faire* approach to the issue of youth unemployment which was reflected in their lack of concern over the high rates of young unemployed school leavers and the depressing prospects for their alumni. St Hilda's did, however, engage the services of private enterprise, in the form of the London Chamber of Commerce and Industry (LCCI) which had approached the school with regard to recruiting trainees for its programmes. The Youth Training Scheme that they organised, 'Enterprise Training South', was situated in their South London training centre.

The representative sent by the LCCI, Mick Payne, was a young, enthusiastic man who introduced himself and the programme employing professional, hard-sell tactics. He began by telling the (pre-examination) fifth year that 'this was a good deal . . . think about it; you don't even need exams to get on to a scheme'. He explained that the schemes they offered trained them for 'white-collar work', to which a boy called out, 'You mean, to become a priest?'

Mick Payne went on to explain that the LCCI had decided to participate in YTS because they felt that the bad publicity surrounding it of 'slave labour' and low wages was not altogether true. The scheme they were offering was for office and clerical staff, and after a period they would put trainees in contact with companies or firms (mainly LCCI building or development concerns) for a job placement. However, Payne explained that they could not guarantee terms and conditions during the trainee period as this was not built into the programme. For example, the provision for part-time release to do study was discretionary, as were hours. But he attempted to reassure them that, 'We do use our political muscle to get you the best deal, in that way you can be sure we care.'

The one aspect of the scheme that was fixed was the wage which, as Payne explained, was £25 a week, adding, 'Well, at least it's better than being on the dole. And remember you do get bonuses like lunch and travel allowances.' After outlining the terms and conditions of the traineeship which, in spite of the professional delivery, still came across as being heavily weighted in the interests of the employer and not the trainee, he urged: 'Go on, give it a try. See a work experience officer and get on a scheme you like. Organisations and companies need young people and young people need us. I can assure you most get a job afterwards.'

However, the pupils remained largely unresponsive and unimpressed. Though many of the pupils were disruptive during the talk, the black girls were generally attentive. At the end of the session the questions directed at Payne clearly made him feel uncomfortable. The black girls took the lead. The questions they asked, however, differed in content and direction from those of their white female peers. The black girls were concerned to know exactly what the scheme could offer them; what prospects did it offer, and could they really be assured of a job? They found his replies unsatisfactory, as one girl explained:

> I hope to be a secretary. What I asked him was how do I know that you will not make me make cups of tea and call that training and then after tell me, 'Bye, thanks a lot, nice to know you'? All he says, well, there are no ways of knowing, but he don't think it true . . . that ain't good enough. [sic]

Unlike the boys,[5] the white girls were openly critical of Mr Payne and his scheme. The following extract from the discussion gives a fair indication of how the fifth form felt in general about YTS.

> *Question (white girl)*: You says the individual person is important then why can't I get into a bank in the ordinary way, but I can as a YTS trainee for the same job? If you say you are so important then you should be judged as a person, not by the scheme you're on.

> *Answer (Mr Payne)*: But you are important; that is why schemes are there to help you find out about work.

> *Question (white girl)*: I think your schemes are exploiting us, you say it's for training but I have a friend who worked in a shop on a scheme, she got twenty-five pound a week but this other girl, her friend, well, she was getting eighty pound for the same job, and just because she weren't on a scheme.

> *Answer*: Well, no. You must remember that you are being trained; the other person, the friend, was not. You are in a better position

to be offered a job with that employer in the end when you finish the scheme than if they didn't know you and what you can do. Work experience is so important with regard to promotional prospects, you could advance so high in a job.

Question (white girl): Yes, that's OK, but I have a friend, she was a supervisor . . . then someone with 'O' levels came in above her with no experience.

Answer: I'm sure that is an exception and not a rule.

Question (black girl): What guarantee do we have that we will get a job when we finish, then?

Answer: Ah well now, it is up to you to inform yourself as to the success rate of the 'trainers'. Ask to see files, ask questions, we need young people and most get a job.

Question (black girl): Could you tell us if we can learn about computing?

Answer: Well, as far as I know very few have had experience in this field, as I said we are aiming for mainly clerical and office skills.

Question (white girl): Has unemployment gone down since YTS began?

Answer: Well, no. . . .

Question (white girl): So what's the good of it then? And what use is it if we ain't gonna get a job after slogging it out on YTS?

Answer: Forget unemployment figures, you can get a job if you really want one, the figures won't tell you that though. Don't worry about unemployment.

Question (white girl): But now with YTS all the jobs are taken, so there is no jobs for us lot leaving school. It forces us to go on a scheme to get a job, we are being forced to do a job for twenty-five quid, not what we should be getting, eighty quid or whatever.

Answer: But I will say to you again, you must think of the training advantage . . . . For the employer the main reason for offering you the job, and let's be honest, is that it is firstly a good way to get good recruits. But there is another reason. Believe it or not, not all employers are bad. They do have a social conscience, they want to do as much as they can to ease the unemployment situation.

Question (white boy): So why ain't unions doing schemes then? I heard they can sack you when they want . . . there ain't no unions or nothing.

Answer: We at the LCCI will monitor and check you. But you have a point, there is no real security. But remember you also have to commit yourself for twelve months to one employer.

In conclusion, the way YTS was introduced varied according to the different perspectives that each of the schools had towards their pupils. St Theresa's, while giving sound but traditional further and higher educational advice to the academically inclined students, siphoned off low-ability pupils into low-level courses which eventually led to YTS schemes. St Hilda's, on the other hand, with its casual approach to pupil performance, did not have such an obviously structured programme. At this school they were inclined to leave the fate of the pupils of whatever ability level to 'market forces'. The YTS input into both of the schools was characterised by a lack of innovation and encouragement to their young black female pupils to seek non-traditional occupations, thereby rein- forcing the low expectations of the pupils and the school.

MAKING CHOICES: THIRD-YEAR SUBJECT OPTIONS

In the third year of secondary school the pupils have to choose the subjects that they would like to take in their final examination in the fifth year. The choices made by these 14-year-olds are of crucial significance in structuring the future career paths of the students. This early requirement to specialise affects the future career of a pupil in many ways. It can lead to exposure to or restriction from certain areas of the school curriculum which can make a substantial impact on shaping a pupil's success or failure in her academic performance. The importance of the third-year option choices was recognised by the schools themselves, as the following message to parents indicates:

I look forward to seeing you all on the 13th March. The careers officer and school careers advisor will be available at the school on the evening to give you advice on how option choice affects career prospects and to give you a realistic assessment of career opportunities.

(St Hilda's Newsletter, issue no. 40, p. 2)

A teacher summed up the circumstances under which most pupils have to make their third-year subject choices: 'It is hit or miss really. It is left to chance. In this day and age it can't be left to chance' (Mr Higgins: D&T teacher and third-year tutor, St Hilda's).

Both schools had a similar procedure for determining the options of the pupils. It was a system that as Ms Wright, head of year for the third years at St Theresa's, outlined, 'greatly depended on the performance in a particular subject, especially with regard to the sciences.'

The head of St Theresa's, Ms Grey, acknowledged the role of the teachers in the decision-making process when she issued the following warning to her staff: 'Sometimes teachers have strong objections to having a girl in her group. If a girl is in your group it is *her* choice and you must talk it over.'

The head of Careers, Ms Wallace, indicated that in other less direct ways a teacher could influence the choices being made by the girls. She explained: 'When girls make their choice the fact of liking a teacher is very important to them.'

Despite their apparent awareness of their role, the teachers, rather than attempting to redress this issue, continued to hamper the career choices of the girls, as one teacher explained:

> The girls should realise the importance of not being able to get on with a member of staff. They must find out who is going to teach them and what group they are in or else there will be trouble. It can be like rubbing sandpaper if they don't get on.
>
> (Ms Smith: Mathematics teacher, St Theresa's)

This teacher clearly felt that it was the responsibility of the pupil to side-step certain subjects in order to avoid confrontation rather than its being up to the teacher to make the effort to reassess the situation.

'Liking a subject', as well as liking a teacher, was another criterion upon which young black women made their subject choices. The head of year for the thirds at St Hilda's, Mr Robbins, explained that this was due to the fact that at this age the student had little experience or knowledge on which to base their career choice. This was supported by the pupils themselves who, upon being asked what future careers they could see themselves in, gave a limited and predictable range of occupations. This was hardly surprising, since the third year had only been scheduled for two terms of careers instruction, most of which in both schools they had missed due to time-tabling problems and lack of teachers. HMI had recommended that formal careers instruction need only start at the age of 13, when 'the eyes of the young need to be opened to wider possibilities' (DES 1973).

As a reflection of the inadequate service these pupils had received by the third form, many young black women stated their reason for choosing a particular career was because it was something that they had 'heard about'. For example, a common response was that it was a job that their mother, aunt or sister did, or that they had seen it on TV. The simplicity of their decision-making process (and its consequences) is illustrated in the following statements:

> I really want to do the child development course. I'm looking forward to it because I like children and look after my brothers and sisters.

> I'd like to be a PE teacher because I'm good at sport.

> I'd like a hospital job. Physiotherapy or something. My sister does hospital work so I've heard of physiotherapy. I read something about it and I like first aid too.

> I think I'd like to do pharmacy. I saw a film about it. But it will mean that I will have to do all three sciences and I don't know if they will let me.

> My parents have a business. But I don't want to do it. My sister made them angry because she wanted to do dance and art. I don't know what to do.

The poverty of the girls' knowledge about labour-market opportunities was apparent. On the whole they had traditional female expectations of work[6] (marriage, however, was not a criterion), and made their subject choices accordingly.

A third-year tutor explained the many pitfalls young black women encountered when they made choices based on very little background information with regard to what a specific job actually entails: 'Many want hospital careers because they get it into their head, physiotherapy, radiographer and so on. But when they hear you need physics, they soon drop the idea.'

Marcella Browne (1981) observes that there are two factors that affect female occupational choice processes. The perception of the opposite sex's response to career development (that is, an awareness that boys do not like girls to work or do better than them) and the anticipation of future adult roles (motherhood and marriage). For the older black girls in the study these two criteria were less of a consideration. However, the younger black girls, who had far less experience of life, were more apt to base their career decisions upon romantic images of their future roles and relationships shared by the wider culture.[7] For example, marriage and the desire for economic security through masculine support was evident among the third-year girls and was in sharp contrast to the response of the fifth-year girls. Ms Wallace commented on a third-year class: 'You can see how unconsciously being a girl creeps in on every level of choice and career aspirations, well, you heard, all they want to do is have babies and marry someone rich and famous.'

In spite of the staff's recognition that these 'gendered' choices were negative and regressive, the counselling which the third-year pupils underwent when making their option choices did nothing to counteract this process.

In spite of the schools' limited attempts to involve them, parents, on the whole, did not feel part of the choice process. In both schools the attempt to involve the parents was a cosmetic gesture. The previous year at St Hilda's the third-year parents' evening during this period had been cancelled. This year the school failed to issue an option booklet to every parent in order that they could discuss their child's choices at the parents' evening. When met with parental objections, the school's excuse was 'because of curriculum changes'. At St Theresa's the attitude towards the role of the parent was made clear when a teacher remarked, 'We were fortunate this year the parents' evening coincided with the option choices.'

Parents indicated that they felt that they were presented with a *fait accompli* with regard to the subjects their daughters would be studying. Option forms were sent home for parents to inspect and sign, but only after the teacher had counselled the pupil on what to do. When parents were consulted, the teachers, from a position of superior knowledge, often persuaded them what was in their daughter's best interests. In this regard parents, such as Anita's mother, were willing to leave matters in the hands of the teachers, saying: 'I don't really understand what going on all the time or what they saying, is the way they says it too' [*sic*]. Other black parents disliked the situation and so avoided coming to the schools. As one parent said, 'I feel unwelcome when I do come, I don't trust them but then I'm not able to argue with them, they'll just go and put me in my place' [*sic*].

Another set of factors influencing career options were time-table restrictions and individual school course requirements. Often pupils could not take up their chosen subject because it clashed with another. In both schools subjects were organised by subject 'block'. Sciences rarely coincided with other sciences but overlapped with the humanities curriculum, therefore making it impossible to do a certain science, for example chemistry, with a specific non-science subject like history. By making a combination of the disciplines difficult, this encouraged pupils, early on in their school career, to choose between the arts or the sciences.

At St Theresa's a maximum of six to seven options was allowed. When making their selection pupils were asked to rank them according to preference, 1, 2, 3, 4, 5, with two reserve choices, 6 and 7. The choices of all the pupils were fed into a computer and a time-table based on subject 'blocks' was worked out. From these blocks the pupils were then allowed to choose one subject. One teacher explained, 'Generally they get their choices, but if not they have reserve subjects.'

The experience of one black third-year girl illustrated the problems of such a system. Caroline wanted to be a nursery nurse; as her teacher explained, 'She has always wanted to be that, she is that type of girl.' Her subject choices were (1) Home Economics, (2) Child Development, (3) Biology, (4) German, (5) English, (6) Geography, (7) History. However, Caroline was advised to drop Home Economics because it was suggested that it was so similar to Child Development and that it clashed with another subject. She was advised to take up Textiles instead. In view of her interests and career choice, for Caroline, who wanted to do home economics, this was an unsatisfactory choice.

School policy also impinged on the girls' ability to choose what subjects they wanted. One teacher explained how the system operated at St Theresa's:

All girls are encouraged to do one language, one science, Maths and English and RE are compulsory . . . . We recommend very bright girls to do 3 sciences, but there are few of those. Geography and Chemistry are very popular this year, even Physics, but that is probably because Ms Grey is a physicist and is keen to promote it.

There were other problems that the girls faced if they chose too many of certain subjects whose syllabi required project work or continuous assessment.[8] If their teachers judged them to be incompetent, girls were steered away from selecting a combination that included too many of these options because of what one teacher called 'practical problems'. She explained:

> Of course when they make subject choices it is not yet decided if they are going in for 'O' level or CSE. CSEs are good, but if some child is put in for four or five CSEs so many projects have to be submitted at once, at the same time approximately. They end up up till all hours of the night trying to complete the work and then you find that even in lesson time they are doing project work for another subject when you are teaching. They have to stay in lunch and rec to complete the work . . . . This always happens to the children who are not aware that they must work on the projects from the beginning and leave it to the end.
>
> (Ms Parker: English teacher, St Theresa's)

Thus the direction which the third-year subject choices took was influenced by a number of factors, of which teacher assessment and the quality of advice were the most important. Within the system of selection, teachers were free to employ their judgement in a number of ways. By their recommendation they could restrict or encourage the take-up of certain options by pupils. The other consideration was the poverty of the careers information that the third-year pupils had received prior to making their choices. Inadequate guidance left these young pupils vulnerable to limited images and ideas of the labour market that reproduced existing inequalities. Without adequate advice the future careers of these young black girls were being determined by decisions that were influenced by the restricted knowledge of both teachers and pupils.

STAYING ON: INTO THE SIXTH FORM

Literature examining the educational characteristics of young black women suggests that they, more than any other group and in particular contrast to their white female counterparts, endeavour to pursue their education beyond the statutory minimum requirements (Dex

1982; Rutter *et al.* 1982; Eggleston *et al.* 1986; *Employment Gazette* 1991).

My study upheld these findings and demonstrated that the majority of black female pupils expressed their wish to continue in some form of full-time education after the age of 16. In response to the questionnaire, 79 per cent of young black women indicated that they would like to continue in their education. Of these young women 65 per cent wished to stay on at school, whereas 14 per cent indicated that they would prefer to leave school and take up a college course. These findings contrasted with the responses of the white girls, 64 per cent of whom stated their preference for staying on (43 per cent at school and 21 per cent at college).

The reason why young black women desire to extend their education is the subject of some debate. Eggleston *et al.* (1986), for example, suggest that one of the main reasons is that young black people, aware of the high rate of black youth unemployment, are attempting to postpone their labour-market entry. There are those who explain the persistence of black women in continuing their education as an outcome of their pursuit of financial and economic independence, especially with regard to their menfolk (Hooks 1983; Fuller 1982; Justus 1985; Moses 1985).

Dex (1983) suggests that young black women who desire to 'stay on' are 'making good sense' of available education and training in response to the negative status occupations and the contracts of their mothers within the British labour market. Rutter *et al.* (1982) offer an alternative explanation. They argue that this phenomenon, particularly among the girls, was a way of counteracting the negative effects of material, economic and social deprivation experienced by a migrant community in Britain, which resulted in the lower attainments of black pupils at their first examination sitting.

However, these explanations did not adequately account for the fact that almost 80 per cent of the young black women in the study wanted to stay on at school. Firstly, there was no evidence to support the findings of those who emphasised the presence of a conscious and universally developed political strategy in the day-to-day decision-making process of young black women. Secondly, there was no evidence to suggest that the material deprivation suffered by the black working classes directly affected the educational outcome of West Indian children, making them stay on longer to get the required grades. What the findings of this study did indicate, however, was that many young black women needed to stay on in order to redress the unsatisfactory outcome of their particular schooling experience. Others who had overcome their schooling experience by re-sitting their examinations were found to be engaged in the normal process of staying on in order to get the necessary grades for further or higher education.

That the schooling experience is particularly weighted against the academic success of young black women has already been established in previous chapters. This factor, when considered in the light of the positive orientation of working-class West Indians to the merito-cratic ideal, explains the necessary persistence of young black women in their pursuit of educational qualifications.

It was found that 82 per cent of young black women in the sixth form at St Theresa's at the time of my fieldwork investigation were doing re-sits in order to get the required grades to further their educational or vocational careers. Of the 15 young black women in the lower sixth, 13 were re-taking some or all of their CSEs or 'O' levels.[9] In the upper sixth, five of the seven black girls were still engaged in re-sits, while two had gone on to their 'A' levels. At St Hilda's all of the five black girls in the sixth form were involved in re-sits while at the same time engaging in other courses (including one or two 'A' levels).

Because of the importance of the 'age factor' in the recruitment process of the youth labour market, it should be recognised that the girls' strategy to maximise their potential by staying on longer was not always a plan that worked out in their best interests (Lee and Wrench 1983). Employers, as well as both private and YTS appren-ticeships, show a preference for younger but more qualified youth. They look to qualifications being gained early (that is, at 16) and at one sitting, and have been found to be less interested in the number of 'O' levels gained over a longer period. Leaving school at 16 has, therefore, a definite advantage over leaving school at 18.

It is important in our discussion to consider the impact of the changing role of the sixth form. The current role of the sixth form was characterised by its inadequate definition. On the one hand, the sixth form retained its old function, a place for nurturing higher educational aspirations; on the other hand, it was seen, with the growth in youth unemployment, as a site for delaying labour market entry. However, the young black women in the sixth form, the majority of whom were there because of the need to re-sit their exams, were not concerned with either of these two aspects. The consequence of being caught up in the contradictions created by these two distinctly different roles was that the black girls received little advice or information to fulfil their needs and requirements (namely, qualifications that were not of use for higher education, or suitable to enhance labour-market opportunities).

Both the quality and orientation of the careers advice offered, and the non-academic input into the sixth form curriculum, reflected the school's ambivalent position with regard to its role. While there was an apparent increase in the number of vocational courses being offered, there was no complementary development of advice and information. Careers advice still largely focused upon its 'prospective university material'.

There was much evidence to suggest that the role of the sixth form was changing. The sixth form in recent years had broadened its scope, offering many pre-vocational and vocational courses, as well as other non-'O' and 'A' level programmes. This change was not always welcomed by the staff, many of whom found it difficult to accept, as one teacher explained: 'They only go into the sixth form because they can't do anything else. They come back because they found out that there is nothing else to do and we are safe.'

There was some evidence to suggest that the sixth form was engaged in a process of 'mopping up' school leavers who were either undecided as to future careers or under-qualified for them. For example, at St Hilda's several pupils who had failed to get their required CSE grades had returned to the sixth form after the summer to do a City and Guilds course (no. 365), which was a general foundation course. One girl, when asked about the course, replied: 'I don't know what it is or what I shall be doing really, they haven't told us much. . . . '

Mr Gavin, the tutor in charge of the course, explained that it was a vocational preparation course with work skills. The pupils, he said, get day release from the college for work placement. It was for those with some CSE passes who were not sure what to do but were not yet ready to leave.

This increased interest of the schools in encouraging pupils to stay on into the sixth form can partly be explained by the budget arrangements the school had with the ILEA. The sixth-form budget is adjusted according to the number of pupils in its sixth form. Ms Carter, the sixth-form mistress, explained: 'There is a problem if we lose too many pupils to college courses. The school loses money and staff. So it is in our best interests not to over-inform them, that's Ms Grey's direction anyway.' Ms Grey did indeed support this policy as she explained in the Quinquennial Review: 'We wish to encourage girls at St Theresa's to return to school after the age of 16, rather than to depart to college.'

Likewise, St Hilda's had a positive recruitment drive aimed at encouraging the fifth-year leavers to go on to the sixth form. The fifth form, in contrast to the information they received on other career matters, were given several talks about the sixth form as well as each being issued with an attractive sixth-form prospectus.

Many of the young black women expressed dissatisfaction with what the sixth form was offering them in terms of vocational courses, and indicated that they would opt for a college future in this respect. One black girl remarked: 'They ain't doing you any favours, you know. They only want us for the money that they get for us. That is why they want you to stay. But I ain't staying long if I can help it.'

Despite their apparent wish to stay on, their choices in the sixth form reflected this disenchantment. It was observed that many of the girls, upon completion of their re-sits after the first year of the sixth form, drop out. The decision to leave indicated that these girls were seeking their vocational training elsewhere.

The vocational courses that were available were limited by the schools' resources. St Theresa's had just introduced BTEC and TEC vocational courses in keeping with the changes around them, and had 'widened the scope of their secretarial course to suit the greater range of ability of girls following the course' (Quinquennial Review).

St Hilda's offered RSA and City and Guilds, and had links with local colleges for pupils to do such courses as 'Motor Mechanics' and 'Catering'. They also offered what they called a 'Basic Clerical Package' and an 'Engineering' and 'Community Care' package, the last two being CSE-orientated.

An increase in the number and type of courses available to the sixth form was partly due to the setting up of 'consortia'. The consortium arrangement came about in 1981 in response to the apparent need for rationalisation of sixth form resources in the face of falling school rolls. It consisted of several neighbouring schools collaborating so that a pupil might take a course offered by any one of the sixth forms in the consortium. Both St Hilda's and St Theresa's had the co-operation of three other schools.

The efficiency of the consortium arrangement was called into question by St Theresa's Quinquennial Review. It noted that pupils in the consortium suffered from the lack of communication between the schools. There were a number of practical problems that resulted from the lack of co-ordination that this produced. Time wasting, time-table and record-keeping problems, differences in examination boards and even hostilities between rival gangs based at the various consortium schools – which included incidents of sexual harassment – were highlighted. In spite of these fundamental problems with the consortium arrangement the schools themselves recognised the need to overcome them if the sixth forms were to survive.

It was recognised at St Theresa's that careers advice suffered because of the consortium, as it was not included as part of the sixth-form curriculum. However, this was only one of the factors contributing to the poor quality of careers advice in the upper school. The sixth form in both schools, despite increases in vocational courses, retained an assumption about the extraneous need for careers advice.

Careers advice in the upper school was largely non-existent. There was no time-table allowance and, as the Quinquennial Report and prospectus of the schools pointed out, it was up to the pupils to seek their own advice. What was clear, however, was that such advice that was available was orientated towards those who wished to pursue a career in higher education, at a polytechnic or a university.[10] St Theresa's illustrated this primary objective of the information service it provided when a central feature in the prospectus under *Sixth Form Careers* noted: 'Mrs Carter advises 'A' level students and has a responsibility for UCCA forms and arranging interviews with the careers officer.' St Hilda's also shared a similar perspective with regard to careers advice in the upper school. In the prospectus it explained that 'Careers advice is always available. In addition to the careers staff attached to the school we enjoy the help of a specialist careers officer who advises those taking 'A' levels.' The message is clear, careers advice is only for those taking 'A' levels and not for those undertaking vocational preparation.

In conclusion, those who entered the sixth form in order to re-sit exams, and not to take up either a career in higher education or a vocational programme, received little support at this crucial stage in their decision-making process. These black girls who chose to 'stay on' into the sixth form so as to secure the necessary qualifications to proceed in their career were found to be caught up in the changing role of the sixth form. As a consequence, the sixth form failed to offer the appropriate information to assist these young women to make informed and non-traditional choices concerning their occupational destinations.

For young black women, the proposals put forward in the government's 1991 White Paper on post-16 education and training (*Guardian*, 21 May 1991) appears to do no more than consolidate the existing shortcomings of the tertiary education system. The White Paper's superficial and political endeavour to abolish the academic and vocational distinction in post-compulsory schooling will do little to redress young black women's clearly expressed concerns about the qualifications they perceive as necessary in order to gain a fair chance in the labour market. As their aspirations towards academic qualifications illustrate, young black women acknowledge, as do most educational commentators (Ball, *Guardian*, 28 May 1991; *Independent*, 5 June 1991), that the labour market is still overwhelmingly determined by the demands and old-fashioned prejudices of the employer, which have been left unchallenged in the government's sweeping reforms.

THE EFFECTS OF SITE AND SITUATION ON OCCUPATIONAL CHOICE

An important factor affecting the quality of institutional resources available to young black women is the site and situation of the schools and agencies to which they have access. The schools that the young black women in the study attended were located in disadvantaged inner city areas of London. This location has implications for the standards of schooling that the pupils who attend such schools receive. For example, Pettigrew (1986), referring to research at Johns Hopkins University, suggests that the location of schools in mainly black areas decreases the employment opportunities for blacks to move out of traditional areas because predominately black schools (1) reduce networks and the 'strengths of weak ties' (Granovetter 1973); (2) reduce 'mixing skills' among blacks (that is, blacks tend to choose predominantly black work situations; and (3) reduce chances of college admission into better-resourced white colleges (i.e., activate prejudice against admitting pupils from certain schools without a tradition of admission).

Although site and situation do have important influences on information, access and resources, there are those who argue that the occupational disadvantages experienced by young black people can only be understood in terms of their geographical location in the inner city (Cross 1986; Wilson 1987; Rex 1988; Smith 1989). The assumption of these 'spatial' studies is that *all* blacks in the inner city experience the effects of 'urban blight', such as rising unemployment and the decline in manufacturing industry, in much the same way.

For example, Cross and Johnson (forthcoming), calculating on the basis of male heads of household, suggest that within the inner city West Indians are skewed towards the bottom of the socio-economic hierarchy. In contrast, they argue that in the outer areas of the city a greater proportion of the ethnic minorities resident there are to be found in skilled, non-manual, professional and managerial social and economic groups.[11] It is clear that the specific employment patterns of black women are not seriously considered in such an analysis.[12] For if they were, it would become clear that while black women's employment opportunities are affected by the process of urban decay, the characteristics of their occupational location cannot be understood only in terms of such forces.

While the initial location of migrants in the labour market in the inner city was determined by job availability and government policy, the subsequent employment opportunities for young black women in London have been structured by the sexual dynamics of the labour market. This is demonstrated by the fact that the employment opportunities available to black women are markedly different from those available to black men. In London 53 per cent of black women are to be found in non-manual occupations, compared to 20 per cent of black men (Brown 1984).

Not only are black women in London to be found concentrated in the non-manual sector, but they are specifically to be found in the service industries, the major employers being the local authorities and the National Health Service. Black men, in contrast, are more likely to be employed in manufacturing and transport and communication sectors of the economy, mainly as skilled and semi-skilled workers. The differences in employment patterns among male and female black migrant workers appear to have influenced the career choices being made by the second generation. Young black women entering the labour market feel they can more readily turn their aspirations towards the non-manual sector than the young black men who, like their fathers, have been traditionally locked into the rapidly declining skilled and semi-skilled occupations.

When the occupational aspirations of the young black women in the study were investigated, it was found that they were generally choosing community and care-orientated professions. The girls were determined to stay in London[13] and take up work as welfare officers, probation workers, teachers, social workers, child–care workers and nurses. Various types of office work, from computing to administration and secretarial work with the large local authorities and other branches of the welfare state, were also regarded as feasible occupations. In short they were opting for jobs that were traditionally done and known to be available to black women in the inner city and that were now essential to the servicing of their community.

An analysis of the employment patterns of the two boroughs in the study, Lambeth and Southwark, reveals that the distinctive aspirations of the young black women could be influenced to some degree by the local labour-market opportunities that are open to them. For example, women were most likely to be found in Southwark employed as clerical and office workers (20 per cent). This was followed by service, sport and recreation workers (18 per cent). Manufacturing, where the majority of men were to be found, only made up a small proportion of female employment (5 per cent).

In conclusion, the evidence presented here suggests that the black female work force in the inner city is locked into a different occupational sector from that of black men. As a consequence of a racially and sexually segregated labour market, black female workers experience different opportunities (that is, access to various types and levels of non-manual work) and difficulties (female school leavers have a higher rate of unemployment in the inner city)[14] from their male counterparts. Partly because of limited access to information, young black women do tend to choose the sorts of jobs that were known to be available to them. In this regard the location of the schools in the inner city can help explain, in part, the initial job choice of some young women.

CONCLUSION: ACCESS, INFORMATION AND ADVICE

Willis (1983) suggests that to emphasise the failure of agencies and services in the career process is to fall foul of the 'matrix of inappropriate middle-class logic'. He explains:

Studies of the transition from school to work, which might have made the connection between the school, social system and the world of work, have simply been content to register a failure of the agencies and rational policies – derived basically from middle class preconceptions.

(p. 99)

Willis's vitriolic attack on those who suggest that careers agencies play an important part in the shaping of young people's careers is based on his finding that 'In terms of job choice it was the "Lads" culture and not the official careers material which provided the most located and deeply influential guide for the future' (p. 106).

Willis claims that the process responsible for reproducing labour-market inequalities and class differences can be illuminated not by an investigation into the delivery of careers information, but through an analysis of the reproduction of culture:

> Counter-school culture blocks, or reinterprets, the formal information concerning work with which it is saturated. All official communications about careers and work are importantly filtered through the group. By and large what might be termed as denoted messages from teachers and careers officers are most heavily filtered . . . information about a job is simply not taken in.
>
> (p. 105)

However, to dismiss the role of information agencies out of hand, as Willis does, is to ignore the fact that many black pupils do rely heavily on the services of official agencies in the recruitment process (Cross 1987a, 1987b). Willis's analysis of shop-floor culture is specific. The internal dynamics he describes that lead the 'Lads' to reproduce their class position is not applicable to the black female context, as some writers suggest (see Fuller 1982).

Young black women are not involved in reproducing their inequalities through their cultural values, but, on the contrary, engage in a process that will, according to their specific rationale, ultimately assist them in securing upward mobility. Within a consideration of this study's assessment of black female aspirations it is clear that the lack of resources will be significant to those who are attempting to secure some measure of upward social mobility through the available channels, and in particular the educational system.

This chapter examined in detail the way in which the quality of advice and access to resources can hinder or assist in the occupational placement process for young black women. It was found that these young black women often chose from a limited range of occupations because they were not given the opportunity to explore other avenues. Not only were standards of education questionable in the two schools studied, which led to a lower level of educational attainment than was possible, but careers advice was also poor and ineffectual. Both the Careers Education Programme and Careers Service were confused in their role, poorly resourced and under-developed. The recruitment to YTS was clearly discriminatory, low-level schemes being aimed at those who were thought of as unemployable. Procedures for early specialisation were not comple-mented by adequate guidance, nor free of teacher prejudice. Infor-mation in the upper school was inappropriate for the needs of the black girls who were re-sitting exams or wishing to go on into further studies. Under these circumstances, and in order that they might further their aspirations and secure some measure of upward social mobility, young black women were placed in a position where they had to rationalise what was available to them.

Thus, in conclusion, and contrary to Willis's position, we can say that the degree to which young black women reproduced their labour-market position was indicated by the lack of any good, positive careers advice. Their cultural values, if anything, assisted them in their struggle to avoid perpetuating their migrant position in the labour market. The question, however, remains as to how far we can claim, from the argument presented here, that a change in careers policy would decrease the level of sexual and racial distinctions in the labour market. This question cannot be answered directly; suffice it to say that inadequate access to information and poor resources did contribute substantially to the reproduction of inequalities.

Chapter 6

Strategic careers

It is only recently that the high and distinctive career aspirations of young black British women have attracted the attention of sociologists and social psychologists.[1] Previously the preoccupation of commentators was with what were considered to be the low and unrealistic aspirations of young black people in general.

Many studies now show that black girls, while choosing jobs ranked high on the social ladder in terms of skill and status, are also selecting distinctively female jobs (Eggleston *et al.* 1986:93). There has been speculation as to why black girls should choose female types of occupation. It has been suggested that black girls do not regard the jobs they select as women's work, challenging the assumption of what is a traditional female job (Riley 1985:66). Others argue that the prospect of men's work is unattractive to women, who see it as dirty, noisy and lonely (Griffin 1985:80).

Some studies emphasise the black mother as the central force in shaping their daughters' aspirations (Eggleston *et al.* 1986:94; Fuller 1982:91). Such an emphasis is inherently problematic as it encourages us to overlook the importance of structural dynamics of a capitalist economy, in favour of the reified 'superwoman' image of the black woman.

If these explanations are not appropriate for describing the social processes involved in shaping young black women's occupational choice, then how can the obvious gender influences that characterise these young women's career aspirations and expectations be explained?

In this chapter I argue that the processes commonly held to structure gender disadvantage are further complicated by the operation of racism. The distinct ideological orientation of working-class, second-generation black women (characterised by a positive tradition of work) also plays a major part in our understanding of the career aspirations and expectations of young black women. The distinctive, high and realistic aspirations of these women are clearly the outcome of a strategy to rationalise the constraints imposed on them by the workings of a racially and sexually segregated labour market.

CAREER ASPIRATIONS AND EXPECTATIONS

In terms of the social class category a job falls into, the career aspirations and expectations of the young black women in the study were indeed distinctive when compared to those of their peers. There were marked differences in job expectations according to the gender and race of the young person, black girls having much higher social-class expectations than any other group. Of black girls 74 per cent expected to find work in either social class 1 or 2 – that is, jobs classified in the professional, managerial and intermediate categories – and many of these young women selecting caring occupations such as nursing and social work were to be found in this group.

Only 11 per cent thought they would obtain employment as skilled, non-manual workers, office work being by far the most popular occupation in this category. Compared to their mothers, 36 per cent of whom were employed as skilled manual workers, only 12 per cent of these girls expected to find work in the same category.

On the whole, young black women seemed the most certain of any group about their job expectations, which is indicated by the small number of girls (2 per cent compared to 19 per cent 'other females') who stated that they 'did not know' what job to expect on leaving school.

When we examine the social class occupational characteristics of the young black men, other interesting patterns emerge. With 27 per cent of the black boys expecting to get jobs classified in the highest category, social class 1 and 2 (professional and intermediate occupations), they also had relatively high expectations of the labour market – however, nowhere as high as their female counterparts. By far the majority of young black men expected to find employment as skilled manual workers (55 per cent – plumbers, electricians and so on). Young black men were clearly avoiding occupations from which they were traditionally excluded, such as non-manual occupations (office work and so on).

When we compare the career expectations of young white women to those of young black women the differences are obvious.

White females had much lower expectations concerning their future employment. Only 35 per cent expected to work as professional, managerial or intermediate employees; almost twice as many young black women expected to take up this type of work.

In contrast to the black experience, however, the proportion of young white women who expected to find employment as non-manual workers was far greater (27 per cent), suggesting that office-type work was seen as an alternative to traditional female 'caring' occupations. Many women who did choose 'caring' occupations chose specific child-care jobs that resulted in their classification in the lower social class group of skilled manual workers (16 per cent classified as skilled manual workers). Another notable difference was that young white women were least sure of their occupational fate: 19 per cent stated that they 'did not know' what job to expect upon entering the labour market.

White male expectations were distinctive. They were secure in the fact that they would be getting jobs as skilled, semi-skilled or unskilled manual workers. A total of 59 per cent expressed their expectations of just such employment futures (45 per cent social class 3 M, 14 per cent social class 4 and 5). The employment expectations of the young white men were the most downwardly skewed in the sample, with only 11 per cent expecting to be employed in any professional capacity.

None of the findings here about the social-class expectations of young black and white people are surprising. Other studies have found similar patterns among their respondents. For example, it has been acknowledged by Fuller (1982), Dex (1983), and Eggleston et al. (1986) that young black women have particularly high expectations of the labour market. Young black men have also been found to have relatively high and 'realistic' expectations about work (Verma 1986; Eggleston et al. 1986). Working-class white girls are often discussed as being confined to the lower end of the occupational ladder (Griffin 1985, Wallace 1987). Willis (1977) and Brown (1987) explain how working-class white males maintain their manual occupational status.

However, what is significant here is the comparative discussion of racial and sexual differences in occupational expectations. The distinctive variations between groups who share objectively a similar class position indicates that a cultural dimension to a class analysis is necessary in order to account for these differences.

It should be noted that the career aspirations of young people embody a different aspect of career choice than expectations. Career aspirations focus on the hopes and wishes of the pupils rather than their more rationally inspired expectations. It is useful therefore to complement an investigation into the social-class expectations of the cohort with an analysis of their career aspirations to see if any differences arise.

The NCDS Survey (Fogelman 1983:273) suggests that there was little variation between the aspirations and expectations of their cohort. However, my findings showed that while this was true of the young black women in the study, it was less so for the other groups. The aspirations for the others were markedly higher than their expectations.

Although young black women appeared assured about being able to fulfil their hopes when they entered the world of work,[2] young black men were less confident.[3] In contrast to their expectations, the aspirations of the young black men were much higher. Whereas only 27 per cent had expected to get a job in social class 1 or 2, 46 per cent aspired to attain such occupations. In the previous discussion it was apparent that 55 per cent of young black men expected to be skilled manual workers; however, only 27 per cent of these young black men really aspired to a career where they would be employed as such.

What was interesting to find was the avoidance by young black men of jobs classified in social class 3 (that is, non-manual work). They neither expected nor aspired to these types of jobs (office work, lower-level administrative occupations), which represented an area of employment, due to both racial and sexual segregation of the labour market, from which black men have been traditionally excluded (Brown 1984).

Young white women were more likely to aspire to jobs in a higher social class than they expected to achieve. Girls who expected to be employed in a social class 3, non-manual capacity, if given the opportunity would prefer to be working in jobs classified as social class 1 or 2. This preference was indicated by the upward shift from social class 3 (non-manual) to social class 1 and 2 (professional and intermediate occupations) of 12 per cent, 10 per cent of whom appeared to come from the non-manual sector. The lack of confidence that this group of pupils had about being able to secure the occupation of their choice was again reaffirmed by the 12 per cent who, upon being asked what they would *really* like to do, still stated that they did not know.

Young white men showed a similar tendency to aspire to jobs of a higher social class than they expected to get. However, there was a far less marked upward shift in aspirations from expectations than indicated by either their white female or black male counterparts. The majority of these young men expressed their desire to remain by and large working in the skilled manual sector, with 11 per cent of those previously expecting work as unskilled and semi-skilled workers aspiring to join them or secure employment higher up the social scale. Several young men (6 per cent) expecting to find work in the non-manual sector indicated that they would prefer jobs if possible in social class 1 and 2.

The evidence presented here shows the distinctive nature of the career aspirations and expectations of young black women relative to the other groups in the study. The majority of these women both expected and aspired to jobs classified in the highest social-class grouping.

In contrast, young black men, though aspiring to higher social class occupations than their white male peers but lower than their black female counterparts, were less likely to expect to fulfil their aspirations in the job market. Young white women were more likely to aspire and expect to secure employment in social class 3, both in a non-manual and skilled manual capacity, than their black female peers. Though almost as many did aspire to social class 1 and 2 occupations as social class 3 occupations, they were much less likely to do so than their black female peers. Young white men were least likely to want, or expect, a job in social class 1 and 2 of any of the pupils. Their preference for skilled manual work was marked. However, a fair proportion did aspire and expect to be employed as non-manual workers, which was in sharp contrast to the young black men, none of whom indicated that this area of employment was open to them.

THE TRADITIONAL FEMALE OCCUPATIONS

There was a marked tendency among young black women to opt for careers in what are commonly classified as traditionally female occupational preserves. The so-called 'caring' professions – for example, teaching, nursing and social work – were preferred occupational choices. Other white-collar 'female' jobs were also favoured, such as office work, secretarial and clerical positions (in particular, bank jobs and personal assistants were mentioned).

This tendency towards 'female' occupations, also noted elsewhere (Griffin 1985), has contributed to the general assumption that black women are subject to the same forces of sexual stratification as young white women, but with the added dimension of racism (Fuller 1982). While the existence of a sexually segregated labour market does, undoubtably, have an effect on young black women, such assumptions belie the complicated processes that structure black female occupational choice.

An investigation into the occupational aspirations and expectations of the young women in the study revealed a situation in which young black women, highly orientated towards the goal of achievement through educational mobility, were confined to a sexually and racially limiting labour market. Young black women did not seem to be choosing their specific 'gendered' occupations because it reflected an aspect of their subjective perception of their own black femininity. Their choices appeared to be made on a much more rational and pragmatic basis.

When I examined the rationale behind the statements being made by young black women as to why they had opted for certain careers, I found what seemed to be an efficient and resourceful means of maximising their occupational mobility, within the existing constraints. Given the limitations afforded by (1) a racially and sexually structured labour market, and (2) their educational attainment (of which they were under no illusions), the young black women chose 'realistic' careers, those that they knew to be accessible and (historically) available to them.

In other words, the young black women in the study were expressing their desire for upward mobility within the recognisable constraints of accessibility. In the following, more detailed investigation of the characteristics of these 'gendered' occupational choices, the nature of and mechanism by which this 'rationale' operates becomes clear.

1 The caring professions

It is often assumed that girls choose traditionally caring occupations because they are an extension of their socialisation as carers for their family and community (Wallace 1987; Fogelman 1983). For black women it is further assumed that they are involved in these occupations because that is an area that has been historically considered to be black women's work (Parmar 1982). Although there is truth in both these statements, they do not provide an adequate explanation of the subjective occupational rationale evident among the young black women in the study.

'High' status (and culturally prestigious) caring jobs, such as social work, teaching and some types of nursing,[4] were not so much regarded as preferred careers because of the qualities inherent in the job; namely, 'helping others'. These jobs were regarded more as a means of obtaining occupational mobility via the route of educational qualifications (necessary in these vocations), within the confines of traditionally acceptable 'black women's work'.

The aspiration towards professionally qualified, caring occupations was particularly true of young black women from working-class backgrounds who were found concentrated in the average and higher-ability ranges in the schools, as the following examples illustrate:

> I have chosen to go to college at the end of the year because the job I want to do only happens at college and not at school. The course I want to do is social care and lasts up to 2 years. At my age now I would not go into a job because the payment at 16 is disgraceful. So if I go to college for 2 years then I would leave and get a job after I know that I am qualified.
> (Dianne, aged 17; father: welder; mother: cook; ability high)

Dianne's statement clearly shows that her decision to do social care is based largely on the fact that for her it offers the opportunity to go on and enhance her financial status by increasing her occupational mobility. Educational qualifications are seen as part of that process, and for black women social work is a known and safe option in which to strive for such a goal.

The girls, however, did not dismiss outright the caring aspect of the job. They often articulated their covert desire for mobility via further educational qualifications within the overt context of 'helping others': Sharon's ambivalent statement illustrates just such a position:

> My plans are to stay in education until I get my 'A' levels. Then I plan to go to college to become a qualified social worker as I enjoy working with other people to try and solve their problems.
> (Sherry, aged 16; father: stripper and cleaner, London Regional Transport (separated); mother: education welfare officer; ability high)

The motivation for achievement through educational qualifications is, for young black women, reflected in their choice of social-work jobs. The occupations they chose always required a course or several courses of rigorous professional training. Thus, when we consider the reasons why the girls aspired to high-status, caring jobs, they were in effect expressing their meritocratic orientation within the constraints of a racially and sexually divisive educational and economic system.

Often the girls' statements indicated that they saw these high-status, caring professions not simply as a vehicle for self-advancement, but also as a means to obtain some degree of community advancement. They regarded these jobs as affording them opportunities to create better conditions for black people in Britain. Marion, who wished to become a probation officer, was one such young woman to articulate this more politically motivated sentiment:

> There are so many black people in prison because of the police. There is a need for black people in social work as so many black people have it hard . . . what I would like to be is like Harriet Tubman, a black woman who had determination.
>
> (Marion, aged 16; aspiration: probation officer)

Nevertheless, many of the girls' statements, though couched in altruistic terms, still retained a basic motivation: that of securing some form of educational and hence occupational mobility, as the following example shows:

> I hope to get a good job. . . . I would not like a low grade job. I would like to work with the community. I hope to do law or social work, something to help the black community.
>
> (Eleanor, aged 16; mother: playgroup attendant; father: absent – died of cancer when Eleanor was 13 years old – ability high)

Not only were the young black women in the study rationalising their educational and labour-market opportunities, but there was also evidence to suggest that this was true of their mothers. Many such mothers of girls in the study who were already involved in the caring professions, especially nursing, or some other aspect of the service industry, were often to be found engaged in processes of re-training or to have already re-trained.[5]

In an effort to secure better employment and enhance their prospects, the black mothers were becoming involved in the higher-status, specialist caring occupations, such as youth and community work, education welfare work, and so on. The tendency to try to move from one caring job to another in order to enhance one's prospects seems to suggest that something more than just the caring motivation was involved in the decision-making process. If caring was the only reason for choosing an occupation, then there would be less likelihood of finding evidence of this desire to change jobs among the older black women. These women were clearly using their existing knowledge and experience of the labour market in order to initiate, within the restrictions imposed by a lack of information about alternative strategies, some degree of upward mobility.

This resourcefulness aimed at maximising opportunity was, among the mothers, not dissimilar to that being illustrated by their daughters, and adds further weight to the argument that the caring professions were (though not always perceived as such), a means of gaining occupational mobility for working–class blacks.

As with the high-status caring occupations, lower-grade (in terms of objective status and pay) caring occupations, jobs often with a geriatric or child-care emphasis, also had important meaning for young black women. These working-class girls, who were to be found in the lower end of the ability range in the schools, would specifically opt for these types of caring professions – professions that, in contrast to the higher grades, required (1) lesser qualifications (for example, nursery nursing did not need the same entry qualifications as social work); and (2) were jobs that the first-generation, migrant women were known to have been successful in obtaining (such as SEN nursing – see note 4).

These lower-grade, caring occupations were a realistic means of maintaining status for young black women not only of working-class origin but also from a middle-class background. They fell within the range of limited and acceptable female occupations open to black women; those black women who were aware that they did not possess the necessary entry qualifications to go on to Further Education college courses such as the CQSW (for professional social work training).

That these specifically recognisable, female caring jobs (nearly always orientated towards child-care) were a way of maximising educational attainment and occupational status is illustrated by the case of Annette. Annette gave as a reason for choosing a job as a nurse simply 'because I like the job they do'. She had no real idea of what the job entailed or why she wanted to do that specific job, only that it was the job she wanted. Annette came from a large family, with four younger brothers and sisters, no father was present and her mother worked as a cleaner in a West End hotel. For Annette, who was placed in the lower-ability stream in her school, nursing was not an unrealistic choice to make. It encompassed mobility, status and the likelihood (based on her knowledge and experience of black women's work) of her achieving such a career.

Vivian chose nursing for slightly different reasons from Annette. She, like Annette, was in the lowest stream of the fifth year (verbal reasoning score, 3). However, Vivian had a different family background. Her mother did not work and her father was a 'businessman'. Thus for Vivian, who enjoyed a middle-class, black family life-style, nursing did not represent occupational mobility quite in the same way as it did for Annette. However, it did mean the realistic maintenance of status for Vivian within the context of her ability. Once again, the historical tradition of black women being located in this profession influenced her choice, in that it seemed a plausible and attainable occupational goal.

The rationale for choosing other types of lower-grade caring occupations, such as nursery nursing, was not dissimilar to that of nursing itself. Quite simply, these occupations were not subjectively regarded as of low status by the young women who aspired to these child-orientated careers. They were seen as challenging, obtainable, fulfilling careers by working-class girls, particularly those from the lower end of the ability scale of the school. Child-care was regarded as a full-time career, not a temporary stop-gap before having their own family. Nor was looking after children perceived as an extension of their femininity, as was the case among many of their white counterparts. Given all the limitations, nursery nursing and child-care vocations were a realistic and pragmatic aspiration, as Louise's statement indicates:

I want to go on to the YTS doing training for a nursery nurse of the age group 3–4 and 5-year-olds. I want to do this because while I am at home I take care of this age group [sister's children] and have experience of feeding, changing, etc. I also have child development in school to help me in my career.

(Louise, aged 16; ability low–average)

2 Office work

Whereas the increase in white-collar opportunities for black women has been the focus of much attention in the literature analysing the black condition in the USA (Farley 1984, 1985; Farley and Bianchi 1985; Wilkie 1985; Simms and Malveaux 1986; Geschewender and Carroll-Seguin 1990), it has been far less central in the analyses of black employment opportunities in the UK. However, from the statistical evidence provided by the Labour Force Survey (*Employment Gazette* 1987) and the PSI survey (Brown 1984), it is clear that white-collar work, a growing sector that provides much 'women's work', is also creating employment opportunities for black women.[6]

The availability of jobs in this area of the economy has had a marked impact on second-generation West Indian female employment patterns. There has been a change among the second generation, reflected in their occupational aspirations. Compared to their mothers, who as migrant women were confined to either intermediate occupations (social class 2; for instance, nursing) or skilled and semi-skilled work (social class 4; such as cooking, factory work and so on), these young women had a wider degree of choice. However, this opportunity for increased access must be regarded in the context of female youth unemployment: young black females between 16–24 years old have one the highest rates of unemployment.

Like the caring occupations, office work was related to the level of the girls' educational attainment as well as to their social background. Skilled, but mainly 'processing' office work, such as typing, secretarial, word processing and clerical tasks (especially working in a bank in that capacity), were careers aspired to by young black women of working-class origin. Girls, particularly with parents in unskilled or semi-skilled occupations, and who were also defined as lower achievers in the school, saw these jobs as a means of getting on within the constraints that surrounded them. As Maureen explained:

> I want to get a reasonable exam result for my job. . . . I want to be a secretary as it is a good sort of job to have.
>> (Maureen, aged 16; mother: dinner lady; father: currently unemployed (used to work in a chocolate factory); ability low)

Thus these types of office jobs were regarded as upwardly mobile choices for young women whose migrant parents had been, or still were, located in the often unpleasant, badly paid, sector of unskilled/semi-skilled manual labour in the UK. The office jobs chosen by the girls were, in contrast, clean, and as one girl put it, 'in a nice environment', and they also offered a reasonable salary as well as a degree of status among the black community.

These jobs were also pragmatic choices, for not only did they present attractive prospects to the girls as far as pay and conditions were concerned but they were also attainable in terms of the necessary qualifications. As Lisa explained:

> I would like to work as a bank clerk or secretary. . . . I would not like to do anything that is low grade which I never dream of doing.
>
> (Lisa, aged 16; mother: clerical officer, Local Authority; father: mechanic; ability low)

While many girls chose the processing type of office occupations, others opted for higher-grade, administrative office work. These included such jobs as legal secretary, personal assistant, bookkeeper, and local authority positions that required specialised training, like housing officers. Choices such as these were made by young women with a low to average school record whose parents, and mother in particular, were to be found in the higher social-class occupations (such as teachers, nurses, social workers).

These administrative jobs were often chosen as careers in contrast to the care-orientated occupations of their mothers and sometimes sisters. Such positions were seen as occupations that they could realistically aspire to within their educational limitations, and yet offered the prospect of Further Education college courses, status and a bold departure from their mothers' often difficult experiences in their welfare-orientated occupations. Several young black women were influenced more directly in their career choice towards administrative occupations by a parent, most often a mother, who had also achieved a high-grade office position in her working career. However, this pattern was only observable in a minority of cases.

Office work, it is argued, reinforces the oppressive nature of female employment (Cockburn 1987), by embodying sexist images of women that, even though they can be seen objectively to degrade and oppress them, are subjectively aspired towards by many women (Griffin 1985). However, office occupations were not chosen on the basis of 'glamour', the reflection of their femininity, or because they offered a chance of meeting a husband, as it has been suggested. Unlike their white peers, young black women regarded office work as providing status and prospects in a field previously denied them because of racism. In contrast to the pervasive image of office jobs as degrading women's work, and which are often seen as only temporary positions before marriage, Rose describes her perception of a career in office work:

> I would like to be a private secretary to a legal firm (solicitors) or in the civil service. . . . I wouldn't like to be in a job that was boring, tedious, unsatisfying, and low paid. Or any place they treat women like dirt, especially black women. . . . I want to be an independent lady. Not dependent on any one, particularly a man.
>
> (Rose, aged 17; mother: senior administrative assistant; father: civil engineer; ability low–average)

Rose was under no illusions about why she wanted her office job.

3 Skilled and semi-skilled manual women's work

Hairdressing and catering, although objectively classified as low-status women's work (social class 4), were not subjectively regarded as such by the relatively few black girls in the study who chose these jobs. As with the case of office work, these jobs were not chosen primarily because of the specific forms of femininity that grooming and cooking implied, but also because of the opportunities that such jobs provided for girls faced with very limited occupational choice.

These manual service occupations were selected by girls who had the lowest attainment records in the school, girls who quite often expected to receive, and in fact received, none or very few, low-grade CSEs. These girls often indicated that Child Development and/or Home Economics was the only CSE they hoped to pass and in both schools were placed on YTS courses geared towards such occupational destinations as child-care. However, in spite of this divisive influence on their career choice and their often unhappy and unsuccessful school record, these young black women still adhered to the ideology of credentialism. They remained positively motivated by the possibility of further educational opportunities outside their present schooling experience. As Angela explained:

I want to leave school, then I want to go to college then I wouldn't might do [*sic*] catering.

> (Angela, aged 17; mother's occupation: 'done work gose to collage' [*sic*]; father, works in shop; ability low).

Some girls, while attracted by the image of the job, still emphasised the training element, as the following example illustrates:

I want to go to college and study professional hairdressing and modelling as it is something I always want [*sic*] to do.

> (Paula, aged 16; ability low)

Her mother being a domestic worker in a hospital, Paula's aspirations toward modelling, about which she was emphatic, must be seen in the light of her knowledge and experience of unskilled black women's work, a fate easily hers without any qualifications.

The nature of this motivation, which could so readily be labelled as a form of escapism, must be qualified. The choice of 'female-type glamour' jobs was not, as is commonly believed, a form of female fantasising on behalf of the girls in the study. The young black women were not projecting into the job any feminine desires they might have about their womanhood nor were they attempting to reaffirm their sexuality. These jobs offered the hope of success and a modicum of achievement without requiring many educational skills, which, although they were well aware these had been denied them, they still struggled to achieve.

This is clearly illustrated by one particular case. Tony, a bright and articulate girl who had been in 'care' all her life (two foster homes and three children's homes), stated her preference for an acting career. While this occupation is not classified as unskilled or semi-skilled work, it would be easy to assume that her reasons for choosing acting were based on escapism from the harsh realities of her experience. She had been put in the lowest ability rank, had a reputation for being difficult and disruptive, and had gained very little from her schooling.

Nevertheless, Tony seriously aspired to an acting career as a realistic and pragmatic (and for blacks acceptable) means of expressing her obvious learning ability, so far untapped and unrecognised by the teachers in her school. She complained bitterly that drama was not a subject offered in the school curriculum, saying: 'All int to do is go into acting.' She had no illusions or regrets about what some would consider her 'deprived background'. In response to the question 'Who would you most like to be like?' she wrote, 'NOBODY ONLY TONY SMITH!'

It is interesting to note that 'working in a shop' was never mentioned as a career in this occupational category of women's manual work. It was, however, a popular choice among young white women of a similar social and educational background. In contrast to their white peers, shop work was considered by the black women as low-status temporary work, not suitable for committed participation in the labour market.

NON-TRADITIONAL AND NON-GENDERED FEMALE OCCUPATIONS

I now turn to an investigation of the tendency to choose 'non-gendered' occupations which, although apparent among young black women, was less obvious among their white peers. 'Non-gendered' occupations, in contrast to 'female' occupations, are jobs that are not traditionally considered to be 'women's work', but are also jobs that are not in practice the sole preserve of males either, even though they are clearly dominated by men. These jobs not only include many of the traditional and established professions such as doctors and lawyers, but also many of the new jobs, such as those associated with computing, precipitated by the restructuring of the labour force, largely as a result of the introduction of new technology and changing economic needs.

1 Special interests: specialised careers

Many young women had special interests from which they wished to develop specialised careers.[7] Girls who had aspirations founded upon their preference for a specific sport,[8] or language, or for a specialised subject such as music, art or creative writing, were confronted with a particular dilemma with regard to the limitations of their schooling.

In order to succeed in their chosen career, they, more than any other group, required the information, assistance, resources and encouragement that only an educational institution could provide. This dependency appeared to put these girls at a severe disadvantage in pursuing their occupational career. As a consequence of the schools' not being able to fulfil the girls' needs satisfactorily, 'luck' more than any other factor seemed to be influential in determining their career. Because the girls' interests were not only beyond the schools' scope and commitment, but also their parents' material resources, it was down to 'luck' if they found out the necessary information to develop a career, 'luck' if a teacher should take a special interest in them and 'luck' if they received any recognition for their ability and achievements.

Thus, more than any other factor, what guided the young black women who wished to pursue a specialised career was their particular sense of determination, as the following examples show. Avril, who was 18 years old, had a special interest in drawing and painting. She was from a single-parent family. Her mother, a nurse, had died when she was 13, and Avril lived with her father, who was employed as a painter-decorator. More than anything else Avril wanted her career to be built upon her love of art, as she explained: 'I want to study art, and then to make some sort of practical use of it. . . . What I'd really like to do is study art therapy . . . but whatever I do I'd like to be best at it.'

Avril, on her own, had researched her career path thoroughly. She told of how she had found 'little joy' in the school's career advice programme, but had finally found a suitable art course at Goldsmiths' College. In order to meet the entry requirements she was staying on at school to do her 'A' levels. Because her father supported her fully and she was a determined, organised young woman, Avril was able to overcome the odds, and in particular the indifference of her school, in order to pursue her interest and career successfully.

Unfortunately, Avril's case was not an uncommon experience. Another young black woman with a particular capacity for art also found little encouragement from her school. Frances did not only encounter indifference but also disbelief from the teachers at her school when she expressed her serious ambition to go into fashion design. The attitude of the school towards her wish to be a 'designer' was that it was unrealistic, particularly for a black woman. Frances, confident and convinced of her own ability, persevered in her chosen ambition. She, like Avril, had to make her own enquiries, and eventually applied for a course at the London School of Fashion, from which she has since graduated.

Similarly, Dianne, without any encouragement from her school, successfully pursued her career in interior design at the London School of Furniture (she subsequently graduated with a very good pass and has since gone on to further studies). 'Luck' appeared to play a major role in determining the careers of the young black women who wished to develop, from their special interests, specialised careers. To have 'luck' as a central factor in shaping their future is both an uneconomic and unfair means of rewarding the enthusiasm, interest and skills shown by these girls.

An example of the schools' indifference towards their black female pupils who desired non-traditional careers was seen in the case of Tony (see pages 129–30). Tony demonstrated the frustration of many black girls who felt that they were not being taken seriously. She wanted an acting career, but did not have any other sources for information and support than those provided by the school, and was unable to fulfil her ambition or put to good use her obvious energy and enthusiasm.

In contrast to the young black women who displayed a particular interest in academic and/or artistic careers was the experience of the girls with athletic and sporting inclinations. These girls were not only encouraged by the staff, they were also favoured. It was not uncommon to hear them referred to as 'polite', 'hard-working', 'talented' and so forth). However, as Laurie experienced, there were constraints put upon her which limited her ability to exploit her interest and skill to its full.

Laurie was the school's top tennis player. She excelled in the sport. Her career aspiration was to be both a sports journalist and, as she put it, to 'play the professional tennis circuit'. But although her obvious ability in the sport was widely acknowledged, the teachers held quiet reservations (expressed only in the staffroom) regarding her ability to succeed in such a competitive field. These were articulated in such statements as 'she's good . . . but you know . . . it's very competitive out there', which was founded upon their understanding of tennis as a sport for the privileged: a sport in which black people do not have a 'tradition'.

Among the teachers there was an objective hierarchy of 'respectable' sports for black people, and tennis was not one of them. Laurie, it was commonly held, was over-confident in her aspiration to become a professional tennis player and, unlike other, less skilled white girls in her year, received little real encouragement. With the best of intentions the teachers attempted to divert her from a career path that, in their estimation, was futile. As far as they were concerned, it required money and social status, none of which Laurie had.

It is clear, then, that a major influence on young black women with 'high' occupational aspirations was the teachers' subtle preconceptions regarding the acceptability of black girls in various subjectively defined, 'socially elite' occupations. This is further illustrated in the case of those girls who displayed a particular interest in creative or journalistic writing.

Young black women who wished to develop their writing skills into a career – one girl was already writing for a local newspaper – curbed their aspirations in the light of their knowledge of the difficulties of succeeding in this profession if one was black. Many girls stated their desire to be 'black journalists', not always because of a feeling of political commitment, which some expressed, but rather because they felt that they would not be accepted as anything else within the media.

When it came to encouraging the girls to go into journalism, and especially with regard to 'mainstream' rather than 'black' journalism, the teachers remained indifferent, offering little or no practical advice on such matters as college courses, believing too that journalism is a 'tough profession', particularly if you are black. The girls, it was clear, had their ambitions restricted, not only because of their own preconceptions, many of which were shaped from hearsay, but because of the limitations imposed by others about what was a feasible career route for black women.

In conclusion, there seemed to be a belief among the teachers that to recognise the presence of specialised skills and special interests among young black women was to condone 'elitism'. This was clearly a misguided interpretation of black achievement. The discouragement of enthusiasm and ability was justified among the staff with the rationale that 'they will only be disappointed if they strive too high'.

2 Higher educational aspirations and the professions

Like those young black women with an interest in developing specialised careers, those who chose the 'professions' or opted for a degree course found little encouragement from their school either in terms of attitudes or in information. They too owed much of their educational achievement and career orientation to personal motivation and perseverance. Most of the girls who chose professional careers were from working-class backgrounds. As Jackie, a working-class black girl who had secured eight 'O' levels and was now taking three 'A' levels, explained:

I would like to do a degree in psychology, preferably at a poly-technic. . . . I expect to be a psychologist or [have] some career in the science world. Something professional.

(Jackie, aged 18; mother: cook; father: welder)

The types of careers many of these girls chose were distinctive compared to the traditional professions their indigenous white (nearly always middle-class) peers aspired to. The young black women in the study were choosing degree courses leading to tradi-tional, often male-dominated professions such as the law, medicine, accountancy, business management and journalism, and there was even one pilot, whereas their white counterparts, who unlike them were mainly middle class, opted for degrees that would enable them to become linguists, teachers or, most popular of all, selected degrees not directly related to any profession, such as literature and 'the arts'.

This observation is supported in the findings of the 1983 National Child Development Study (Fogelman 1983:275). The evidence of this research suggested a pattern among white women graduates (nearly always of middle-class origin) of choosing 'female-type' pro-fessions such as teaching, or high-status caring professions, especially social work and hospital careers. In contrast, the NCDS suggested that the boys, very much like the black girls in my study, were more likely to opt for such traditional and prestigious professions as medicine and the law.

There is a general concern that not enough black women enter the teaching profession in Britain. As my evidence suggests, not many black women make a conscious choice at 18, if they have the ability and determination to attempt a degree, to enter the teaching profession. They are more likely to choose more lucrative profes-sions if given a choice. For historical and other reasons degrees in education (including the PGCE) are not such an attractive propo-sition to black girls who have managed to reach this level in their academic career.

The orientation of the young black women in the study towards their professional qualifications was very different from that of their white counterparts. With their educational background it was logical for these high achievers to wish to extend their education and, at the same time (as we have already witnessed among their black peers who aspired to the 'caring professions'), to maximise their credentials within the given constraints of a rigidly defined and male-orientated professional hierarchy. Ruby's direct and determined statement when considered in the context of her family background reveals just such a rationale:

> I would like to stay on at school and do three 'A' levels. After I would like to get into a university and get a degree in law. I intend to be a barrister and practise in London.
>
> (Ruby, aged 16; father: clerical worker at Gray's Inn (works with QCs); mother: nursery teacher (retired))

Ruby was influenced by her father's job and saw this profession as a realistic way to maximise her educational ability. It entailed status prospects, social commitment and, not least, some degree of financial reward for her effort.

What was clear in the study was that the black girls did not want to undertake a higher degree for the sake of 'self-exploration', nor for the luxury of extending their education. Nor, as Tomlinson (1983b:79) points out, did they wish to pursue their university career because they saw themselves as either 'victims or superwomen'. Higher educational opportunities offered the prospect of both enhancing their career status and their capacity to earn a good wage. This did not mean that the girls were ruthlessly pursuing a professional career at the expense of all else. Many girls did express their commitment to helping others through their own achievements, as the following statement suggests:

> I want to be a doctor, not necessarily a doctor in a surgery, but active as in helping the people who have most need of it. Back home I would like to help them, especially those who cannot afford treatment because most doctors are private and private means expensive.
>
> (Levine, aged 17)

However, the lack of career advice for girls wishing to enter the professions or wishing to take up a higher degree meant that many bright young women made their choices from the traditional professions or found themselves insufficiently advised when it came to deciding how best to apply their educational skills, a situation that the following example illustrates:

> I know that I do not want a job just yet. I want to get into a degree course somewhere, but I haven't . . . I mean I don't know what to do.
>
> (Frances, aged 18)

Other girls did wish to choose more specialised professions but were aware of the possible prejudice they could face. In the following case, although Floya was from a middle-class background, she was aware that her prospects could be hampered by racism. She opted, not for her chosen career, but for a career that she knew, from experience (her father was in that profession), to offer slightly less resistance.

> I would love to study archaeology or the classics . . . but that's way out there . . . I'll never get into Oxford and all that, you must be kidding, [in posh accent] la, de lala [all laugh] . . . but I'd like to do a BA degree in business studies, accounts and that, then go for a certified or chartered accountant degree.
> (Floya, aged 16; father: certified chartered accountant, mother: playgroup leader)

The desire to minimise racist experiences had the effect of cancelling out any innovative attempts in non-traditional professions that had not been tried and tested. Racism in this context (and in the context of the other careers so far discussed in this section) can be regarded as an external pressure which ensured the reproduction of certain professions from one generation to another.

3 New technology and aspirations towards non-traditional female occupations

There is a common assumption that young black women 'naturally' gravitate towards non-traditional 'female work' (Griffin 1985). Their desire for woodwork and other conventionally defined 'male' subjects at school is often cited as evidence of this uniquely black female tendency (Riley 1985). Their relatively higher uptake and enrolment on 'trade' and access courses, leading to plumbing, electrical and carpentry training, is also used to indicate this trend (Cockburn 1987).

However, the evidence presented so far in this chapter suggests that the majority of black women do opt for what can be described as the more traditional black women's careers. Nevertheless, there was some evidence that black girls were far more likely than their white peers to move willingly into traditionally male occupational preserves. Why should this be so? To date, the explanation for this phenomenon has centred on an argument which suggests that this willingness is a form of resistance; a conscious statement of 'black womanhood'. However, in my opinion, the willingness of young black women to undertake traditionally male work is the outcome of two aspects that are related to their orientation to work.

Firstly, there was no evidence of any cultural constraint that inhibited a woman from aspiring to any occupation that she felt competent to train and undertake. Secondly, all the evidence so far suggests that young black women are primarily motivated in their career aspirations by the prospect of upward mobility. A job, therefore, is an expression of the desire to move ahead by means of the educational process. The belief in the promise of a meritocracy and the rewards of credentialism spur black women on to take up whatever opportunities that may become available and accessible to them, especially opportunities that entail a chance to increase their further educational qualifications.

An example of the determination to succeed whatever the odds can be seen in the case of Marion. After undertaking a three-year course in social care at the local college of Further Education (Brixton), Marion was unable to secure a job. The local college, however, offered Access courses. These courses enable those without the necessary and appropriate qualifications to enter into specific vocational training or academic institutions. Marion, a resourceful and serious person, decided that rather than joining the ranks of the unemployed, she would enrol on an Access course that would enable her to become an electrician. Her decision must be seen in the light of a course being offered in an accessible college.

The question arises as to whether Marion and the other black women really wish to do electrical work, and whether this demand gives rise to the courses. Or, as seems more likely, was the accessibility of such a course and the prospect of gaining further credentials the reason for its uptake?

With the recent growth of new technology, jobs needed to service this industry have become available. However, the mystique of the computing world has not deterred some young black women from venturing into this male-dominated preserve. These young black women liked the type of work and saw it as an opportunity to express their ability, regardless of gender. They were not put off by its image, as Veronica explained: 'I would like a job in medical research and computing. . . . I want to be a person who can be accepted at any job he or she wants.'

Another example of young black women's confidence to move away from traditional female occupations, as well as, in this case, black occupations, was illustrated by several girls (and boys) who expressed their aspiration for a career with the police and in the British armed forces. They were convinced of their choice. They did not feel that they should be excluded from aspiring to these professions just because of the army's racist and sexist track records: after all, as one girl pointed out, she might be black but she was also British.[9]

The police and the army were considered in two different lights. Many girls expressed their dislike of the police, an opinion based largely on experience (32 per cent). However, one girl desired and eventually did go on to join the police. The army, by contrast, was seen as far more remote in terms of its oppressive function and role. The girls who chose this career saw it more in terms of a good solid career.

A job in the armed forces offered the girls an attractive proposition: the possibility of ascription, security, excitement, travel and, most of all, the promise of equal recognition for equal achievement among men and women, as well as among black and white.[10] It was clear that it was the image more than anything else that attracted the girls. They identified most strongly with the latter aspect of the army career; that is, the hope of equality. For, despite the cultural orientation within the black family that suggests the relative autonomy between the sexes, black women still have to struggle for even a modicum of respect and equality within the work place.

The girls who opted for an army career were from the average to lower ability range within the school and were aware that they could look forward to a less fulfilling career than that which the army could offer, as Trudi explained:

> I would like to join the WRNS or the army as a cadet. I would not like to work in any kind of an office . . . what I want is an interesting job that pays a good wage and that I like to do and will get respect for doing.
>
> (Trudi, aged 18; mother: works in a hostel for women; step-
> father: teacher, head of physics in a secondary school; ability,
> average, in sixth form has obtained four 'O'levels and two CSEs)

FOUR YEARS ON: AMBITIONS FULFILLED OR DENIED?

The investigation so far has focused on what the young men and women said they think or hope will happen to them when they leave school and enter the world of work. Four years after the initial survey, a questionnaire was sent to all the black male and female pupils in the study.[11] In spite of their realistic and strategic career choices, the test of time revealed a disturbing picture of unfulfilled aspirations and wasted potential.

Staying on

Of the young women who replied to the questionnaire 77 per cent indicated that they did for some period 'stay on' at school after the age of 16. Of these a majority (70 per cent) were involved in the process of re-taking CSE or 'O' levels or were engaged in other academic pursuits, such as doing their 'A' levels in order that they might go on into continuing or further education.

When they left school 45 per cent of these girls did go on to continuing, further or higher education. Many, though not all, took up a social care type of course. Only 10 per cent stayed on to do re-takes with the intention of entering the labour market directly upon leaving school. They were re-sitting in order that they might enhance their prospects in the job market (most entered into higher-grade office work, such as that of a civil service clerk) or secure the required qualifications to enter a particular profession (like the police).

The remaining 30 per cent who stayed on were involved in the vocational courses offered by the sixth form. The take-up of the secretarial programmes was especially notable.

The Youth Training Scheme (YTS)

Of all the female destinations 29 per cent were YTS placements. A disproportionate number of these placements were office work, often low-grade clerical positions. Several girls worked in private companies (for example, a record company, a bank and a solicitor's office): the others were employed by large public employers (Lambeth Council, County Courts, and so on).

What was clear about these placements was that they did not reflect the girls' choices. Most of the girls involved in this type of office work had indicated as their original aspiration a 'community' or 'care' placement. Many of them had taken up school courses in order to go into 'socially orientated' occupations, as the following case illustrates.

Louella wanted to do a YTS course in nursery nursing and had taken up (and passed) Child Development (along with four other CSEs) in order that she might do so. However, she was given an office placement, and as the following account of her subsequent and unsatisfactory experiences of the YTS shows, she has since spent three years attempting to secure her chosen vocation in 'community care'. She is currently employed as an assistant caterer (cook).

In 1984 after I left school I went to Brixton College. Then I went on holiday for a few months in Jamaica. After I returned back to London from my holidays I went on a YTS scheme as I had taken all my interviews before I left.

This was a one-year computer course in Kennington. On this course I also did typing, data-base word processing and communication skills. When I went on my work experience I was a VDU operator for Sandell-Perkins which took me on full-time. I was there for a little while becoming an experienced VDU operator.

All during this time I also had an evening job as assistant caterer in Covent Garden. I left Sandell-Perkins as I was not happy with things such as the pay, especially as I was getting double the money for my evening job.

I went back to college part-time to do a 'community care' course at Vauxhall.

I have now left college after passing my exams and I got a pay rise from the evening job which I also do two full days. Move from parents' house. Settled down. I hope one day to get a job in community care [sic].

The young black women who had stated their aspiration as office work, and in particular secretarial work, were on the whole the most successful of all the girls in fulfilling their aspirations. These five girls did their vocational training at school or at college (for example, 'Sight and Sound') and then sought and secured work almost immediately, as the following typical example illustrates:

Marcia
   1984: Sixth form St Hilda's: secretarial course
   1985: 1 year BTEC at South East London College
   1986: Junior Secretary for R. Mansell Ltd
   1987: Ditto

On the other hand, several young women with good academic credentials, who did not state their aspiration as office work, appeared to enter this field of employment because of its availability. It was clear that these three young women, in terms of their qualifications, were under-employed. For example:

Janet: Aspiration, to go to university and study business.
- 1984: 2nd year of 'A' levels (still at school) (2 'A' levels)
- 1985: Work for a solicitor as a clerk (London Buses, clerical assistant)
- 1986: Still with London Buses as clerical assistant
- 1987: Still with London Buses, promoted to assistant buyer

Social welfare and caring occupations

In contrast to office work, none of the 12 pupils in the destination survey who had aspired to a 'caring' profession (that is, teaching, nursing, social work and so on) had by 1987 successfully secured a position within their chosen field. The destinations of those wanting to pursue social work careers fell into three categories:

1 those who wanted to do YTS care-orientated courses but were placed on office-work programmes;
2 those who went on to college to train specifically to be in a 'caring' profession but have since been unable to find appropriate employment;
3 those who were still at college engaged in the lengthy process of qualifying for a professional career.

We have already examined the first case, that of thwarted ambitions, as the experience of Louella (above) showed. However, as disturbing as the case of Louella were the four instances where young women, after qualifying, were unable to find appropriate employment. The experience of Marcella provides an example of one such case.

Marcella's ambition, contrary to her teachers' advice, was to undertake a course in social care with the ultimate aim of becoming a probation officer. For two years she studied social care at Brixton College while working part-time on the weekend to supplement her income. In 1986 she secured a temporary training placement in a nursing home. However, unable to find a permanent postion, or indeed any work for which she was trained, she decided to return to college in 1987 to do an electrician's course. She has since had a baby.

The resoluteness with which young black women pursued their careers was apparent. Three young women were still at college, having spent four years without earning any income, in order to achieve their ambition. Denise, for example, stayed on at school to re-take CSEs and to do some more 'O' levels. For the past three years she has been studying social work at the Kingsway Princeton College.

Higher education and specialised careers

Only two girls responding to the questionnaire went on to pursue specialised careers. These girls, both of whom were from working-class backgrounds, had by 1987 successfully completed part of their studies, but as yet had not fully entered the labour market. Dianne, who had left school with six 'O' levels, had been awarded a Diploma in Interior Design and Furnishing from the London College of Furniture, and was now completing a degree in Interior Design and Computer Graphics at Teesside Polytechnic.

Debra had completed a Diploma in Fashion Design from the London College of Fashion (in spite of her teacher's expressed reservations), and was now undertaking an apprenticeship as a trainee designer and pattern cutter in Great Portland Street. These girls provided further evidence of black female willingness to postpone labour-market entry (with the assistance and support of their parents) in order to attain the required qualifications needed for success in their careers.

Business

Though several girls in the original sample had aspired to a career in business, only a few who replied to the questionnaire had succeeded in their ambition. Those who stated that they would hope that doing a BTEC would provide an opening into business were all working as secretaries. One girl, who originally indicated her desire to be a teacher and had gained several 'O' levels and two 'A' levels, had been working in a boutique for three years in the hope that she might one day own her own shop.

Unemployment

Even though no young women actually reported being unemployed, what was immediately apparent was the role the YTS played in successfully masking the lack of available opportunities by effectively postponing labour-market entry. A disproportionate number of young black women were in effect moving from one unrelated scheme to another, as the following typical example shows:

Sonia: Aspiration, nursery nurse.
      1984: YTS 'Newsight' Art and Design course
      1985: YTS introductory course for working with children
      1986: Southwark College City and Guilds for Home Economics and Family and Community Care (2 years' course ended 1988)

Others drifted from YTS to one casual job after another in an effort to avoid unemployment:

Sandra: Aspiration, data proccessing.
      1984: YTS scheme, clerical work
      1985: British Home Stores, cashier, Oxford Street (full-time)
      1986: Tesco Stores, Brixton (full-time)
      1987: Unemployed, 'because I'm expecting a baby which is due in August'. ('I hope this will help you complete your study')

Motherhood

Four years after leaving school 3 per cent of the young black women who answered the questionnaire had become mothers. Entry into early motherhood was not necessarily a substitute for unemployment or poor job prospects, as it is often assumed. Some young women were on the point of completing college courses (social care and word processing), others were still involved with on-the-job training (such as hairdressing), while others had secure jobs in various aspects of office work (for example, Civil Service clerk and personnel secretary).

THE CAREER DESTINATIONS OF THE YOUNG BLACK MEN

There were only two replies from the small number of young black men in the study. In contrast to their female counterparts, both had distinctly 'masculine' experiences.

Maurice: Aspiration, electrician.
      1984: Electrical Engineering (Brixton College)

1985: (Apprentice) in Plastering
1986: Ditto
1987: Ditto

Davis: Aspiration, armed forces.
1984: Picture Framing on YTS
1985: HM Forces, Royal Green Jackets
1986: Frozen food department, Jumbo Cash and Carry
1987: Ditto

It should be noted that Davis's Verbal Reasoning score on entry to St Hilda's was highest in terms of Reading and Mathematics, yet by the fifth year he had been relegated to the bottom stream of the year. He was labelled as 'difficult, aggressive and unable to communicate' by his teachers. However, I found him helpful and intelligent. He enclosed the following message with his questionnaire:

> Hi, I don't know if you personally remember me, but I remember you. I hope you are doing well after all these years. I would like for you to keep in touch with me and let me know how you get on with your studies. Davis.

CONCLUSION: FROM CAREER ASPIRATIONS TO LABOUR-MARKET REALITIES

The career choices being made by the young black women in this study were related to their specific experience of the labour market and the educational system. Clearly what these girls were doing was attempting to achieve upward occupational mobility through a strategy that rationalised the various constraints that they encountered.

One major constraint was the existence of a racially and sexually segregated labour market which ensured limited occupational opportunities to young black women. The black girls chose careers that were 'gendered', not so much because of the nature of the job but because that was the only type of work in their experience and knowledge that was available to them. However, in choosing these jobs they used the stated educational requirements as a vehicle for obtaining more or better qualifications, in order to enhance their career prospects and satisfy their desire for credentials. Their willingness to move into 'non-gendered' careers can be largely explained by the combination of the notion of relative equality between the sexes, which meant that there were no cultural limits on attempting to do non-traditional female work, and the motivation to succeed, which encouraged the search for opportunities wherever they were or however they might be defined by others.

In spite of their determination to succeed, the career destinations of the young black women and young black men who took part in the follow-up survey, four years on, were characterised by a distinct lack of variety and scope. For the girls, the overwhelming concentration of employment opportunities in low-grade office work regardless of their aspirations, together with the marked tendency for unfulfilled aspirations towards careers in caring professions, was a clear pattern. The 'masculine' characteristics of the male careers reflect the presence of sexual divisions in the labour market. In general, what was apparent was the wasted potential of both the male and female young people in the study.

Chapter 7

Redefining black womanhood

In the past and depending on who held the pen, black women have almost exclusively been portrayed in terms of negative and regressive stereotypes: 'Sapphire', the overbearing, domineering matriarch; 'Aunt Jemima', the homely, loyal mammy; 'Jezebel', the erotic, sensual temptress (Hooks 1983; Farnham 1987; Gray White 1987). Now black woman are themselves in the forefront of reclaiming their own womanhood, and the arena where their invisibility and misrepresentation is played out is the novel. The novels, essays and poems of Maya Angelou, Toni Cade Bambara, Zora Neale Hurston, Paule Marshall, Toni Morrison, Gloria Naylor, Ntozake Shange, Alice Walker and Sherley Anne Williams, with their powerful celebration of the maternal presence, have been instrumental in opening up the historically and culturally distinct world of black women.[1]

In sociological and educational analysis the attempt to adopt this positive perspective of black female resistance to racial and sexual inequalities has been less successful. As discussed in Chapter 2, the use of the strong role model of the black woman has been found to be problematic when called to account for the experiences of young black women in work and school. Such an emphasis encourages the analysis to look inward to the family as the site for determining success or failure, distracting our attention from the more structural political and economic forces of racism and sexism. Despite appearing outwardly 'progressive', the maternal emphasis has also led to the continued marginalisation of the black male in sociological analysis, first established in the conservative thesis of Moynihan (Spillers 1990).

In response to the problems raised by the maternal emphasis in sociological analysis, which is the strong black female and its complementary partner the marginal male, in this chapter I investigate the presence of relative autonomy between the sexes. To acknowledge that there is a specific form of black femininity among young black women, characterised by relative autonomy between the sexes, explains the different outlooks in terms of school, work and marriage that are evident between cultures.

It is argued that the 'culture of femininity' is the means by which working-class girls come to take their place as dual labourers in the production and reproduction of labour power in a capitalist economy.[2] This theory suggests that young women subjectively rationalise and thus freely choose situations such as marriage and child-rearing which objectively oppress them. With its emphasis on 'subculture' and 'motherhood', this dominant and pervasive explanation of the reproduction of gender disadvantage has offered the ideal framework in which the theory of the strong black female role model could be developed. Indeed, as we have already seen in the work of Fuller and others in Chapter 2, it has formed the basis of the major explanations of black female educational and labour-market orientations.

However, as is so often the case in sociological accounts of inequality, the cultural 'universalism' of the culture of femininity thesis has rarely been questioned. As a theoretical paradigm, this model cannot adequately address the very different nature of the black female experience. This is because as a theory it is in essence culturally specific; making ethnocentric assumptions about the way in which culture, and in particular the role of the family, interacts with the structure of the labour market.

To establish that there is a case for arguing for an evaluation of gender within specific cultural contexts, I shall compare and contrast the second-generation Irish female experience with that of their second-generation West Indian female peers. These two groups of young women offer us an interesting proposition for comparison.

In many ways the second-generation Irish and West Indians share common experiences. Both are the daughters of migrants who came to Britain in the 1950s in search of better opportunities. In this respect both the Irish and West Indians have a similar experience of displacement from what was essentially a rural existence to resettlement in an urban context. Both the Irish and West Indian migrants were the recipients of crude, anti-immigrant hostility by the English, though the post-colonial racism that structured the experience of the West Indians was far more powerful, direct and insidious. Both migrant groups in this study live and work in the same locality as each other, and though they do different types of jobs, they objectively occupy the same (working)-class position.

The fundamental difference between the two groups, other than the obvious one of colour, is the distinct history, culture and hence ethnic identity of each group. For our purposes of rethinking black womanhood in the African Caribbean British context, it is helpful to use the particular cultural construction of one group as a 'control' against the other. In this way we may examine the contemporary characteristics of each of the two distinct cultural constructions of femininity. We begin first with an investigation into the second-generation Irish British experience before we move on to a detailed examination of the second-generation African Caribbean, West Indian experience.

THE CULTURE OF FEMININITY AND THE IRISH BRITISH EXPERIENCE

McRobbie (1978a, 1978b, 1990) whose thesis exemplifies the paradigm of the culture of femininity, argues that appropriate gender behaviour for working-class girls throughout their adolescent years is orientated towards their ultimate *raison d'être*; that is, 'winning' a man and getting married. What directs working-class girls 'freely' into marriage, child-rearing and part-time labour are specific cultural notions of femininity and romance. The ideology of romance, McRobbie argues, transforms the material dominance of the male into an illusion of true love. As such these notions of femininity are not arbitrarily imposed from 'above', but as Willis (1977) describes in the context of his 'Lads', are the outcome of creative negotiation of contrary material and ideological situations.

The acceptance by the girls of their future as home-makers and child-rearers directs them to specific parts of the labour market structured for the female school leaver, a labour market where general conditions and insecurity reproduce female dependency on other sources of material support. As a consequence of the interaction between the cultural construction of femininity and the labour market, most of the jobs available to women involve few long-term commitments, or trade off 'glamour' and the possibility of romance against low pay and poor conditions.

The experience of the second-generation Irish girls in the study suggests that there is no reason to doubt the validity of McRobbie's thesis in particular cultural contexts. Indeed, the actions and beliefs of the girls appeared to support McRobbie's model of the cultural reproduction of the sexual division of labour.

Pupils of Irish descent made up a sizeable proportion of the cohort (26.6 per cent). Like those from the Caribbean, these students were the offspring of parents who had migrated to Britain in the 1950s. Unlike the more recent wave of Irish immigration, this generation of migrants were mainly unskilled and traditional in terms of values (Ryan 1987). The majority of the mothers of this group were employed in unskilled or semi-skilled part-time occupations (such as dinner ladies, cleaners and so on); otherwise they were classified as 'unpaid' (that is, housewives). Fathers were on the whole skilled manual labourers (for example, builders) and unskilled workers.

In interviews, the female contingent of this second-generation Irish population consistently expressed their desire for marriage, having children and looking after a home. For the Irish girls, however, the wish for domestic fulfilment was perceived as incompatible with a permanent commitment to the labour market.

An obvious explanation as to why these girls should juxtapose work with marriage lies in an examination of their (historically unique) attitudes and values. How they articulated their desires gives some indication of how the cultural construction of femininity can be seen, in some instances, to reproduce labour-market disadvantage.

Like the young women of West Indian origin, the majority of second-generation Irish girls also saw themselves as still essentially Irish and not British.[3] They were not only very conscious of their ethnic origins, but as migrants they tended to view their cultural 'heritage' in an uncritical and positive light, as the following extracts illustrate:

> I consider my homeland Ireland. . . . I have been influenced by my parents' background in some sense. Every year my family goes back to Ireland, 'home', as it is called. . . . We are expected to be proud of our Irish background and follow in our ways.
>
> (Mary, aged 16)

> Both my parents are Irish and I have been brought up in an Irish atmosphere. I refer to Ireland as my home.
>
> (Eileen, aged 16)

> I think I am Irish because I have been brought up to believe in God and follow the Irish way of life because it has been handed down to me from my parents. It could be hereditary even.
>
> (Margaret, aged 17)

Ullah (1985:318) argues that girls were more likely than boys to adopt 'an Irish identity', as were the lower socio-economic groups. Indeed, the evidence suggested that these mainly working-class girls did hold strong views on being Irish. Having an Irish identity had important implications for the labour-market participation of the second-generation young Irish women in the study, in that it ensured the maintenance of their traditional values about work and marriage.

What both the indigenous British working-class and Irish migrant cultures in the sample had in common was an essentially 'male-centred ideology'. Beale (1986) comments on this Irish ideological orientation which persists, despite the influence of the Irish women's movement since 1970. She writes: 'The ideology of the family functions to support male-dominated hierarchies, and is another source of continuing oppression for women' (pp.190–1).

Just as McRobbie has argued in the case of 'working-class girls', the traditional Irish ideology of marriage, very much alive among the second generation, does have debilitating consequences for the young Irish women living in the UK. Beale describes what she calls a 'narrow home-based view of the female role'. She argues that it is assumed that once married, a woman and man will adopt fundamentally different roles. It is expected that she will forfeit her right to financial independence and a job, and will always subsume her interests to those of her husband and children.

The girls' career aspirations strongly reinforced their specific cultural concept of femininity. The career aspirations of second-generation Irish girls were noticeably lower in terms of social class compared to the aspirations of their West Indian peers. They frequently chose 'female-type' work such as that of nursery nurses, shop assistants, beauticians, secretaries and so on. Many of the jobs chosen by the girls had less to do with careers and more to do with work. As Kathy, a young Irish girl, explained: 'When I leave school I want to work in Woolworths, then I suppose I'll get married.'

Their statements also reflected their partial and often transitory commitment to the labour market, and illustrated the affirmation of their womanhood through the institution of marriage and motherhood.

I want to be a nursery nurse because I like children and I want to look after them, especially my own.

(Linda, aged 16)

I would really like to be a bution [beautician] because it is a good future for me before I get married.

(Maria, aged 16)

These attitudes were in sharp contrast to those of girls of West Indian origin who, although from a similar migrant background (both parental generations migrated for 'a better life' and left their own countries to get improved jobs and opportunities for their children), aspired to much more demanding careers.

The girls had inculcated in them many traditional values which they expressed. A common view was their opinion on child-care: 'I'll never never let anyone look after my children. You hear all these stories, you know, I'm going to take care of my own' (Linda, aged 16).

The wish for marriage, children and a family life does not necessarily preclude the desire for labour-market participation among all girls. Data indicate a range of differing ethnic attitudes to occupational aspirations and to family life. For example, studies have shown that young Asian women have positive attitudes towards work and the family (Parmar 1982; Bhachu 1986, 1991).

Romantic liaisons were common among the boys and girls. Girls often were found reading romantic comics or books in the lesson, and frequently appeared to be preoccupied with discussions of their own or others' relationships and intrigues. It was also not uncommon to find girls fighting over a boy. During a Maths lesson, for example, a serious and vicious fight erupted between two girls of Irish descent. Apparently hostilities had been brewing for some time, because it was claimed that Mary had 'stolen' Shiobhan's boyfriend. Books, and even chairs, were hurled across the room, to the accompaniment of some rather obscene language and hair-pulling. The girls and their respective 'mates' from rival gangs were oblivious of the classroom situation and undeterred by any threat of punishment they might receive for disturbing the lesson (the teacher turned a blind eye).

By fighting, the girls did not conform to the traditional expectations of what is considered to be 'feminine' behaviour. Whereas some argue that the ideology of romance reinforces the passive acceptance of an oppressive social structure (McRobbie 1978a, 1978b, 1990), other authors hold that that girls often actively assert their position with regard to proprietorial rights over male partners (Wallace 1987). Some commentators on the subject argue that the ideology of romance is an expression of sexual desire and its complex interrelationship with social status (Cowie and Lees 1981). Nevertheless, all the variations of these cultural explanations still conclude that the ideology of romance in the end reinforces the powerlessness of young women's positions.

The experiences of the second-generation Irish girls in many ways did seem to reflect the traditional cultural attitudes of their parents. To some degree the Catholic school environment reinforced and ensured by one way or another the traditional values. However, the migrant situation had introduced many new experiences for the second generation, which had the effect of modifying the traditional modes of thought prevalent among the girls.

A facet of this new social environment was the issue of interracial marriage, and interracial relationships, which often spontaneously arose in interviews. Many of the girls had black (African Caribbean) boyfriends and wanted to discuss the issue.

> My parents would react if I came home with a black boy, but they would not be set in their Irish ways and make me marry an Irish boy. Eventually they would have to accept it. Although I'm Irish I'm not set in Irish ways.
>
> (Geraldine, aged 17)

> In Ireland you don't see many blacks, here you get used to it, learn to live with it.
>
> (Kathy, aged 16)

> I think it's not the colour but what the person is like . . . but my Mum she didn't agree when my sister married a Malaysian.
>
> (Maria, aged 16)

> My Mum said it's OK once they are Catholic. But say if you wanted to live with someone, not marry them, she'll go mad.
>
> (Eileen, aged 16)

Another aspect of change was the fact that many young people realised that they could not bring up a family on one wage. Some, though not all, second-generation Irish boys said that they would want their wives to work. However, this topic often caused a great deal of argument, with the girls especially objecting. Even though the girls openly rejected the idea of working when married, change for the second-generation girls was apparent in their willingness to challenge unacceptable aspects of the present-day youth labour market, such as low wages, unemployment and the YTS programme.

It was an irony that signalled change that many girls who had expressed traditional values with regard to marriage and the family on the one hand, should articulate their dissatisfaction at their economic future on the other.

Several young women of Irish descent contemplated the idea of single parenthood as an economically rational and viable life-style. Some commentators suggest that female-headed families are economically strategic in the context of growing male unemployment (Farley and Bianchi 1985:26). Many girls in my study, both black and white, thought that living together was preferable to marriage, and saw no personal stigma attached to such a decision (although they were aware of parental objections).

Because of the time of migration, the Irish families in the study were by and large quite young. The girls often had many younger siblings. The hardships of the migrant parents, in particular the mothers, had not gone unnoticed by their daughters. Second-generation Irish girls frequently made reference to their mothers' struggle, and to the fact that they did not wish to suffer the same fate:

> It's thankless bringing up children. That is all my mother has done, and you should see where it's got her. Nowhere.
>
> (Ann, aged 16)

> I remember my mother having post-natal depression, so bad. That's how I know how you can feel towards your children. I think marriage, children and all that is a waste.
>
> (Marge, aged 16)

The second-generation girls, by upholding their traditional values, can be seen to be reproducing their unequal labour-market position. The explanation provided by the notion of the 'culture of femininity' seems in this instance to be an appropriate analysis. This notion hinges on the subjectively constructed ideology of romantic love and the acceptance of marriage as a culturally valued institution. However, as the second and third generations begin to question the economic and even cultural rationality of marriage, as in some cases is clearly happening, the causal explanation offered by this thesis for the reproduction of the female labour market begins to break down.

If girls do not accept the ideology that ultimately confines them to certain sections of the labour market and especially the domestic labour market, then how can the perpetuation of a sexually (and also racially) segregated labour market be explained? Would a sexually divisive economy perish with the decline of Catholic morality and the demise of the institution of marriage? Surely not. As the West Indian experience bears out, black women, regardless of their cultural orientation towards the ideology of romance, the institution of marriage, or their objections to racism, still remain confined to a sexually as well as racially organised labour market. The explanation, it would seem, does not lie within a culturalist framework. The evidence seems to suggest the need for a more structural approach; a perspective that takes account of labour-market rationale and highlights the perpetuation of sexual and racial inequalities.

WORK AND WOMANHOOD: THE WEST INDIAN BRITISH EXPERIENCE

Although a general desire for economic dependency prevailed among the young white working-class women in the sample, there was no evidence that this cultural orientation existed among the black working-class women who were interviewed. Whereas *all* of the black girls responded positively to the prospect of having a full-time career upon leaving school, only 80 per cent of their white female peers said they would. Young black women of all abilities and social backgrounds, with a wide variety of career aspirations, reiterated time and time again their commitment to full-time work and their desire for economic independence. Evidence of this positive ideological orientation was clear in the data:

> I would like just like to be an independent lady. Not dependent on any one, especially a man.
>
> (Joy, aged 16; aspiration: legal assistant)

> I don't want to rely on anyone. What I want is a good job as I would like my life to be as comfortable as possible, and have a nice environment to live in so my children can grow up with everything they require.
>
> (Laurie, aged 16; aspiration: journalist)

On the basis of this evidence alone there is little justification for adopting an analytical framework that emphasises the centrality of an oppressive form of femininity, which the prevailing theories on the black female experience clearly do.

The key to why this situation of positive orientation and commitment to work should prevail was provided by the girls themselves.
The statements they made showed that they expected to work just as
their sisters, mothers, aunts and grandmothers had done for generations before them. However, and this is the important point, they
expected to do so without the encumbrance of male dissent. This
meant that the young women did not regard their male relationships,
whether within the institution of marriage or not, as inhibiting their
right to work in any way.[4] It was not uncommon to find among the
girls in the study statements such as these:

> My sister has moved out, got a nice little flat to herself . . . having
> your own place . . . a little job, not getting married, just having
> your boyfriend . . . well, living together . . . no . . . well, popping
> round to see you . . . that what I'd like.
>
> (Debra, aged 16; aspiration: designer)

> Work is as equally important in marriage, or your relationship. I
> don't care if it's marriage or not, whatever, I think it's important.

However, the young women also stated that while they wanted to
work, they did not wish for a repetition of their mothers' experiences. They often spoke of their mothers' work, which was discussed
invariably in terms of hardship and sacrifice. They always gave a
unanimous 'No' to the question 'Would you like to be like your
mum and do the same sort of work?'

> My mum has worked hard to give us things, and to bring us up,
> even if it was shit work. They want to give you all the things they
> never had. . . . I suppose I'll do the same for my children, I mean
> give them what's right.
>
> (Annette, aged 16; aspiration: nurse; mother: auxiliary nurse)

When interviewed on the subject of marriage and women's work,
the young black women in the study agreed that women should
work regardless of child-rearing responsibilities. The following statements were common examples of the sentiments expressed by the
girls:

> . . . even if you have kids you have to work. I sometimes feel
> sorry for my sister's kids. She leaves them with a minder. She
> works in the council or, I don't know, something like that. They
> don't even know who their mother is . . . one day I heard

Damian call the minder mum. I don't want that for my kids. But it's like this, if you don't work what will you do? Stay home and knit? You'll be useless to everybody.

It's important to work and to bring up your family as best you can. If it is your family I think it is your responsibility.

Anita, one of the girls in the study who became pregnant,[5] spoke of her attitude to marriage:

I know for sure that one thing is sure, that I don't want to get married. . . . He says we should, but I feel we are capable enough to make our own decisions and own plans, after all we are adult people. Why does everyone else have to interfere so much? If you ignore others you will be all right but in life you can't . . . marriage, no way . . . we've put in for a flat though. . . . I'm not rushing into anything.

It was commonplace to find bold and positive statements such as this: 'If I don't work I'll go mad. . . . You've got to make something of yourself because in the end no one cares.'

This did not mean, as Riley (1985:69) seems to suggest in her analysis of similar types of statements, that young black girls were pursuing a course of aggressive assertion of their femininity (which in the case of black girls is interpreted as female dominance) at the expense of all else, especially permanent male relationships. Nor, as Fuller (1982:96) suggests, was this the manifestation of a 'going it alone' strategy.

In my opinion what the girls were articulating was a much more subtle ideological orientation than either of these two authors suggest. Unlike their white peers, who had evidently been inculcated in the dominant ideology that women only take on major economic roles when circumstances prevent their menfolk from doing so, the black girls held no such belief about the marginality of their economic participation and about commitment to the family. Providing for the children and the household was regarded as a joint responsibility, as the following statement illustrates: 'I think it is important for a woman and man to work, to both provide for your family is an important thing to do' (Karen, aged 16: aspiration: computer programmer).

The West Indian boys in the study had no objections to their future partners working.[6] They were in full support of their women-folk being gainfully employed, as the following statements illustrate:

My mum, she's a cook and she looks after me and my brother. . . .
I think if I got married, I don't see no difference, I don't see it any
other way really.

> (Davis, aged 16; aspiration: armed forces)

Any woman of mine's got to see about herself anyway, it ain't
gonna bother me, but I ain't keeping no woman, that's for sure.

> (Maurice, aged 16; aspiration: electrician)

You must be kidding! . . . of course she's gonna work. If she don't
work she don't eat! [laughs] Anyway, I ain't getting married.

> (Leroy, aged 17; aspiration: plumbing/central heating)

The boyfriend of one of the young black women in the study, Anita,
who at the age of 16 became pregnant, had a distinctly supportive
and encouraging attitude to her moving ahead in her career, as he
explained:

> A woman must can and must do all she can . . . but I's believe
> having children is very important . . . it's good to have kids young
> and enjoy yourself. . . . You don't have to take time out to do it
> or stop nothing. . . . Of course she will be set back though, and
> we have discussed this, I told her to not to stop school, exams are
> important . . . she can go on to college, you know, yeah, but she
> got to have 'O' levels or she set right back and she'll have to start
> from the beginning, I told her not to stop.
>
> (Winston, aged 23; games supervisor at the local sports centre)

The issue of relative economic and social autonomy between the
sexes should not be confused with the matter of the sharing of
domestic labour or the permanency of male/female relationships, as
is so often the case. That West Indian men do not equally participate
in household tasks is well documented, as is the tendency towards
instability of consensual relationships (Justus 1985; Moses 1985;
Powell 1986). These facts, however, do not affect the matter of joint
responsibility towards consanguineal offspring or children within a
consensual relationship. Relationships which have joint responsibility towards the household, within the context of relative autonomy between the sexes, are a common feature of West Indian life
(Sutton and Makiesky-Barrow 1977: 311–12; Dann 1987:25–30;
Thorogood 1987; Barrow 1988; Mohammed 1988).[7]

The existence of joint responsibility is more widespread than most
sociological commentators of both radical and conservative

ideological persuasions care to acknowledge. This can be argued on several counts. Firstly, as evidence of joint economic responsibility, there are almost equal numbers of black men and black women in the labour market, compared to the relatively unequal situation among the white male and female majority (see Brown 1984: OPCS 1987).

Secondly, although a high incidence of single motherhood is reported among black families (that is, relative to white), the numbers are relatively small in comparison to the incidence of stable conjugal unions that do actually exist in the black community. If these figures are considered in their correct context (that is, not a comparative black–white analysis, as is the convention), family stability still remains the overriding norm among black families (78 per cent compared to 13 per cent is a significant difference – Brown 1984). Thus the majority image of most black men as feckless and irresponsible remains largely a product of media stereotyping and academic misrepresentation (Hoch 1979; Phoenix 1988b; McDowell 1990; Segal 1990).[8]

The relatively high incidence of single parenthood among young black women (vis-à-vis young white women) can more readily be explained within the ideological framework that stresses the relative autonomy and equality between the sexes in the black community. The existence of this ideology encourages women to strive for compatibility rather than economic security (with its attendant values of duty and loyalty) within relationships.

Colin Brown's evidence (1984:37) that single parenthood is not only common among young West Indians but also among older West Indians, indicates that single parenthood should be regarded in terms of a life-cycle phenomenon, with people moving in and out of relationships seeking compatibility and friendship, and, as Barrow (1986) suggests in the case of women, increased economic autonomy.

The young black women in the study did express a cautious yet positive approach to marriage and relationships:

> Eventually I'd want to get married, but you should be like best friends and live together [another girl shouts out, 'You mean platonic'. All laugh].

> Well, things have changed now . . . you can have kids but you don't have to be married. . . . My brother's been together for twelve years and got four kids and they just got married. The girls were the bridesmaids and the boy's a page boy.

The thing that worries me about marriage, right, is that the fact you are stuck with that one person for life . . . because a lot of girls rush 'this is the one for me, this is the one for me,' and all that, and rush into it.

I'll get married when I'm 30 or 35 in the future, after I've done something for myself.

In the study there was no evidence that black men were considered marginal in the lives of young black women. Of West Indian households in the study, to which the girls belonged, 79 per cent had both a male and female adult sharing the parenting role (for white girls 90 per cent belonged to two-parent families). Of the 11 per cent who had only one parent present, 2 per cent were male-headed households, a feature not found among the white families in the study.

Despite the acknowledgement that men in their lives could in the future pose problems, the young black women in the study frequently spoke positively about men and their attitudes. They did so drawing on their own experience and relationships with men, in particular their fathers, male guardians, brothers and uncles.

I don't think really, looking after children hard if the man behave himself. . . . My brother's girlfriend got him under heavy manners right, no back chat, you know, they got three young ones.
(Janet, aged 16; aspiration: secretary; father: bus conductor)

Most men do understand the problems faced by women, I think so anyway. I go to my dad whenever I have a problem.
(Laurie, aged 16; aspiration: journalist; father: telephonist)

My dad wouldn't let me work [Saturday job]. He says it will interfere with my school work, ask him for pocket money instead. I suppose it is for my own good but I feel he's unfair.
(Janice, aged 17; aspiration: social worker; father: painter-decorator)

Since my mum died my dad's brought us up. . . . All he cares about is seeing us do well and going to college.
(April, aged 16; aspiration: art therapist; father: British Rail ticket collector)

Further evidence of black males assisting their partners to stay at work during the crucial and difficult time after the birth of a child is presented in the TCRU Day-Care study (Mirza 1986b). The black relationships in the study provided some of the most unusual and egalitarian forms of partnership. Several men willingly changed shifts to accommodate child-care arrangements. One couple agreed upon a complete role reversal so that the wife, who worked in a bank at a more senior level than her husband, would not lose her promotional prospects. However, in some cases the men did not give much physical help (although they were deemed to be a source of emotional support), mostly because, as one woman said, 'He's always out doing his own thing'. But in these cases the women stated that despite their partners' frequent absences and the problems this caused, the partners did not obstruct their return to work, and if they failed to provide adequate financial and moral contributions, they did at least show affection for the children.

In short, what the evidence revealed was that it was neither the men's absence nor presence that affected the black women's orientation to the labour market.[9] Other factors, specifically the provision of child-care and the accessibility of relatives and the employer, were the crucial variables.

Studies in America (Moynihan 1965 in Rainwater and Yancey 1967), the Caribbean (Smith 1962) and in Britain (Foner 1979) have persistently attributed the relatively high proportion of black women in the economy to the absence of a male provider or his inability to fulfil his role. This pathological explanation of the black family – that has come about from the belief that it is 'culturally stripped', essentially a hybrid of western culture (Frazier 1966; Little 1978) – has failed to acknowledge that black culture has evolved an essentially egalitarian ideology with regard to work, an ideology that, as Sutton and Makiesky-Barrow (1977:323) observe, 'emphasises the effectiveness of the individual regardless of gender'. This argument is supported by the evidence that the proportion of black women in the labour market relative to their white female counterparts is far greater, a fact that is true for the UK and the USA.

The argument that high black male unemployment determines increased black female labour-market participation cannot be upheld; it is a theory based more on a 'commonsense' assumption than fact. Black male unemployment is no higher than black female unemployment. (In the 25–35 age group in the UK, 17 per cent of black women are unemployed, as are 18 per cent of black men. In other age ranges the proportion is even greater for black females; see Brown 1984:190.) The fact that males and females are concentrated in different sectors of the labour market and so have access to different employment (and educational) prospects is not a consequence of choice but rather due to the dynamics of a sexually segregated labour market (see Farley and Bianchi 1985).

The study revealed a notable lack of sexual distinctions about work among second-generation West Indian young people. Many girls said that they did not see any difference between themselves and their male counterparts in terms of their capacity to work and the type of work they were capable of.

I think men and women have the same opportunities, it is just up to you to take it.

Of course women should do the same jobs that men do. If they feel you can't . . . them stupid. . . . Who's to say anyway, it makes me sick it does.

Men should do the jobs women do and women the jobs that men do. There's nothing wrong with men midwives, I think all men should find out what it is like to have a child, it's the nearest they can get to it.

Young black women living in the West Indies expressed a similar point of view with regard to women's work, as one girl illustrated when she stated: 'I think what is good for a woman is good for a man, there's no difference between men and women when it comes to work.'

Further evidence of this trend to refuse to regard certain types of work as the sole preserve of men was shown in the results of the study. Black girls were far more likely to express their desire to do non-gendered work than their white female peers.

This ideological position regarding work expectations cannot be the outcome of a 'female-orientated' tradition (Phizacklea 1983). If it were a female-centred ideology, then it would be difficult to account for the obvious preoccupation many young black girls had for, as one Trinidadian girl explained: 'the need for emotional support and strength from a man, you like to feel he rules, even if he don't.'

The young black women in the study, both in the West Indies and in Britain, often commented on the desire for male companionship. This, and the fact that many women treat men as 'guests in the house' (Justus 1985), has been interpreted as evidence of a male-centred ideology in the West Indian family structure. The description of the black family as having a male-centred ideology is based largely on the evidence of black male non-participation in the domestic sphere.[10]

It is important to note at this point that there seems to be a contradictory state of affairs with regard to research on the status of the woman in the black family, which can result in a great deal of confusion. On the one hand, it has been argued that what exists is a matrifocal, female-dominated structure (Fuller 1982), and on the other hand the family ideological orientation is often described as 'male-centred' (Justus 1985; Moses 1985).

These two fundamentally divergent theoretical interpretations of the ideological dynamics of the black family have evolved as a consequence of the confused interpretation of the two essentially different aspects of family life: relative autonomy between the sexes and male non-participation in domestic affairs. In effect what we are observing in this study is an ideological orientation governed, not by male bias or female bias, but by the notion of relative economic and social autonomy between the sexes.

In home visits to the parents of the girls in the study, the statements by wives and husbands illustrated the existence of a measure of independence between the sexes, as well as joint responsibility towards the family. They frequently related stories and anecdotes that told of their independent, but equal, work roles.

One such example was the case of Mr and Mrs Burgess, who had come to the UK 24 years ago. Between them they had brought up five children, the eldest being the child of a previous relationship of Mrs Burgess. They had both always worked and had an evident pride in their children's achievements (one daughter was a computer programer, another a social worker, while the others, who were still at school, were doing well). They lived on a bleak, run-down, post-war council estate in Brixton. She enjoyed, and got a great deal of satisfaction from her job as a canteen assistant; he found his work 'on the buses' less interesting. Both wages jointly contributed to the family income, although each wage went towards different aspects of family expenditure. He explained in his broad Grenadian accent how he regarded the relationship:

> She does she work, she go in every day, come home every day. She do she own ting really. Half de time I ain't know what she get up to, always going out spending she money on Bingo or some

ting so. I don't min once she leave me alone. . . . I's like to do me own ting too . . . ya know.

Mrs Burgess had her own comments to make: in her equally broad Dominican dialect:

He so lazy, girl. He could sit there all day an' complain. Nothing good enough, well, just sit there then. I does go alone if I want to do anything. . . . I does pick up myself . . . even go by self to de carnival. . . . I's have me work, I's like me work, mind.

The indifference in attitude they now expressed towards each other after many years of marriage should not obscure the relative autonomy each partner enjoyed with regard to their own work and social activities. Despite their disagreements on other matters, neither partner interfered with the other's right to work. For Mrs Burgess her work was and always had been a source of pride and achievement, a realm of experience quite apart from her life at home. She enjoyed talking about her battles and victories in the work place:

When I first came to England dere was so many jobs. I move from one to another. It took me four weeks to find my first job. I work for Lyons. Two pounds fifty I got. . . . I tell you them days a shilling a lot . . . now I'm the only coloured face at work, but I put them in their place, I stands up for myself, I ain't gone to leave because of them few. Me an' the Italian woman wer's the only outsiders so they want us out. They don' like me because I'm better then them, I've got better qualifications them and they's know it, especially that supervisor, that how I got the work. She wanted to get rid of me always shouting at me, but now I've got my friends we get on well, laugh and ting, have a good time, like at de Christmas party.

Considerable independence between the sexes does not presuppose the shedding of social attachments as it can do in other cultural contexts; rather, it necessitates and increases the involvement of both partners in the lives of their families. In spite of their separate economic and social experiences, Mr and Mrs Burgess jointly contributed to the family budget and participated in the upbringing of their children. However, just as each income financed a separate aspect of the household expenditure (see Stone 1983), so too did each partner perform a different parenting role.

They both agreed that 'life hard [*sic*] for the children nowadays', and that it is up to the parents to see that the children do not 'go astray' and were not out roaming the streets, and if they failed and the children were 'bad', then it was the parents who were at fault. They had, especially Mr Burgess, a strong disciplinarian approach towards their children which, it became quite obvious, had alienated the children to some degree.

CONCLUSION: THE CULTURAL CONTEXT OF GENDER

The evidence presented here suggests that the cultural construction of femininity among African Caribbean women fundamentally differs from the forms of femininity found among their white peers, and indeed their white migrant peers. Thus the theoretical arguments about the way in which gender disadvantage is reproduced become inappropriate in the black context. What the young black women in the study were expressing was essentially an ideology that emphasised the relative autonomy of both the male and female roles.

Ironically, the dynamic that has produced this equality between the sexes within the black social structure has been the external imposition of oppression and brutality. African Caribbean societies in the Caribbean and in industrialised capitalist settings have not simply replicated the western pattern of sexual stratification.

Like their parents and grandparents, the young black women in the study had not adopted the dominant Eurocentric ideology: an ideology in which gender is regarded as the basis for the opposition of roles and values. These young black women had, instead, a very different concept of masculinity and femininity than their white peers. In the black female definition, as their statements revealed, few distinctions were made between male and female abilities and attributes with regard to work and the labour market. As to why this particular definition of masculinity and femininity should result in greater female participation in the labour market is explained by Sutton and Makiesky-Barrow, who write:

> the distinct qualities of masculine and feminine sexual and reproductive abilities are not viewed by either sex as a basis for different male and female social capacities. And unlike the self-limiting negative sexual identities the Euro-American women have had to struggle with, female identity in Endeavour [a town in Barbados]

is associated with highly valued cultural attributes. Because the women are assumed to be bright, strong and competent, nothing in the definitions of appropriate sex role behaviour systematically excludes them from areas of economic and social achievement.

(1977:320)

Chapter 8

Family matters

There is a genuine need for a cultural reappraisal of definitions of social class in the UK to be made immediately, not least because of the present misrepresentation of the African Caribbean family in contemporary British class analysis. African Caribbeans living in Britain are no more homogeneous in their class make-up than their white British counterparts, yet they are often discussed as one group.

In the same way that class affects occupational location, access to economic, political and social resources, values and life-styles among the white British population, so too does it influence these factors for blacks. However, just as black families differ among themselves, so too do they differ from white families who have been 'objectively' classified in the same social-class grouping. If black people's class position is defined in terms of their relations to the means of production (that is, ownership), they appear to hold a similar position to that of their white compatriots (Miles 1982). If, on the other hand, their class experiences (life-styles) are taken into account, substantial differences between black and white become evident.

As a consequence of various historical, cultural, economic and social factors, black working-class and middle-class families do have a fundamentally unique experience in the work place, at school and within the family, compared to their white counterparts who occupy 'objectively' the same class position. The racial dimension of the class experience is crucial to an understanding of the distinct aspirations and expectations of black working-class people in Britain. The process of migration has had a significant impact on the experiences, and hence attitudes and values, of working-class West Indians in the UK.

My research indicated that in many West Indian working-class households the woman can often be found in an occupation that may be defined objectively as middle-class (such as social work). However, this fact is largely obscured by the tradition of taking the male to be the head of household. Other distinctions are often misinterpreted because of similar ethnocentric evaluations. For instance, in the life-cycle of the black working-class woman (and sometimes the black working-class man) single parenthood is a not uncommon stage. Furthermore, the presence of relative autonomy between men and women in many black working-class households means that both partners are found to contribute equally to the family income. West Indian attitudes to education are also positive, the meritocratic ideal being a very important determinant of occupational and educational aspirations. Home ownership is also a black working-class aspiration[1] as are a number of other values typically identified with a white middle-class orientation.

A recognition that there is a cultural context to social class does not, as Miles (1984) suggests, render a class analysis invalid. To acknowledge that there exists a black working class with cultural and historical origins distinct from the white working class does not imply that race is subsumed by class. On the contrary, it enhances its meaning, for not only does it incorporate a fundamental recognition of blacks with regard to their relations to the means of production but it also allows a more satisfactory reappraisal of working-class black consciousness.

EDUCATION AND HOME BACKGROUND

A curious state of affairs persists in the study of educational inequality and social class. On the one hand, those studies that investigate the influence of race and gender inequality in education often display a lack of understanding of the fundamental role of social class. On the other hand, studies that address the issue of social class distinctions in education nearly always fail to integrate a consideration of race and gender disadvantage into their analyses.

This compartmentalisation of the various aspects of educational disadvantage seems especially surprising when we consider that they are fundamentally interconnected. For how could an analysis of social class, widely acknowledged to be a major factor in educational inequality, not take into account the fact that blacks and females are the two groups known to suffer the most from the effects of educational disadvantage?

In studies of education and the black experience the consistent misinterpretation of social-class factors is clearly a response to the rigid and ethnocentric interpretation of social class that these studies assume. It is often the case that social class (often referred to as 'parental influence') is not found to be a significant factor in black educational performance. Many studies conclude that the effects of 'ethnicity' override that of social class when accounting for black underachievement (for example, Sillitoe and Meltzer 1985).

When parental background *is* discussed with regard to black educational performance, it is nearly always done so in a negative light. The logical assumption is made that black children from low socio-economic backgrounds must be influenced in the same way as their white counterparts, only worse (for example Swann, DES 1985).

Some studies fail to give a satisfactory account of social class because of its apparent inconvenience to their analysis. For example, a positive appraisal of West Indian class characteristics was incompatible with the Eggleston Report's (1986) emphasis on underachievement and institutional racism.

In a bid to account for scholastic success among black pupils, Bagley, Bart and Wong (1979) makes the assumption that a positive orientation to education is solely a black middle-class phenomenon. But should low socio-economic status always be considered as a reliable predictor of poor educational outcomes?

Clark (1983), in his study of why poor black families succeed, is one of the few researchers to offer insight into what he calls the 'quality of life' in poor black homes. Though his analysis is fundamentally flawed by its emphasis on individual motivation, he does draw our attention to the importance of family disposition, not composition, as a means of explaining the positive orientation of black children from materially deprived backgrounds.

It is a convention in studies that assert there is an important link between the parental background and educational outcome to use the paternal occupational yardstick (for example, Halsey, Heath and Ridge 1980). Likewise, the limited research that exists on social class and educational outcome among black pupils also always uses fathers' social status as a measure of parental background (for example, Sillitoe and Meltzer 1985; Mortimore *et al*. ILEA 1986a). This assumption begs to be questioned.

In order to investigate the effects of home background on educational outcome it was important to examine if there was any measurable influence between the job aspirations of the young black women in the study and their fathers' social background. The findings showed that young black women, whatever the social status of the father, were very likely to aspire to a job of a high social status. This trend was very evident among young women with fathers who themselves were in higher social status jobs. The daughters of men in manual occupations deviated from the pattern only slightly, a small percentage choosing occupations that were classified as non-manual and manual. Those girls with fathers not working in the household, either due to unemployment or because they were not present, aspired by and large to professional and managerial occupations.

Can we assert from the evidence that fathers' occupation influences their daughters' job choice? The data appear to indicate that these young women were not reproducing their fathers' social status, making their choices independently from paternal influence. This was made clear by the fact that many young women whose fathers were in lower-status occupations were aspiring to the same occupational group as those young women who had fathers in the higher professions. Fathers' occupational status could be seen to have some effect when it is observed that girls with fathers in manual occupations were more likely than those from non-manual and professional backgrounds to choose non-manual and manual occupations. However, if the type of work that these jobs entail is investigated, it is evident that they were not choosing to do the same type of work as their fathers. These jobs were regarded as high-status female work and so in a sense represented mobility for these young women.[2]

If the relationship between fathers' job and daughters' aspirations is tenuous, we must then investigate if there is any direct link between mothers' job and daughters' aspirations. It has been argued that the mother plays a central role in influencing the educational attitudes and aspirations of their children (Jackson and Marsden 1963; Hoggart 1957). Other aspects of the maternal influence have also been ascertained. Some studies, for example, investigate the psychological aspect of the maternal influence. Rutter (1981) emphasises its impact on child cognitive development and Chodorow (1979) on 'sex socialisation'. Research on white working-class women highlights the direct and indirect role of the mother in the occupational choice process of girls (Holland 1983).

In studies on the black female a similar case is made for the positive role model of the mother, to account for both the occupational and educational orientation of black girls (Fuller 1982; Phizacklea 1982; Dex 1983; Eggleston et al. 1986). It has even been asserted that the black mother plays a crucial part in the maintenance of educational disadvantage among her children in general (Brewer and Haslum 1986).

What the findings of my study showed was that young black women, whatever the occupational status of their mothers, were more likely to aspire to a high-status career than simply mirror their mothers' occupational experience.

It could be argued that there was some degree of influence of maternal social class, made evident by an increased likelihood among the girls with mothers in skilled non-manual and manual work to choose jobs of that social class, compared with the decision of girls with mothers in social class 1 and 2, who were less likely to take up a career as a manual or non-manual employee. This was further shown by the fact that 25 per cent of the young women whose mothers were in semi-skilled and unskilled occupations opted to do this same type of work.

However, this social class influence can be seen to be marginal in the light of the more marked trend in the evidence that strongly suggests that the aspiration to a high occupational status was being made regardless of mothers' social status, even among girls from a lower maternal social background. That the girls' occupational decisions appeared to be made independently of their mothers' occupational status was further supported by the fact that even girls whose mothers were in social class 1 and 2 (the most common occupational category all round for both mother and daughter) did not necessarily choose the same job as their mothers were doing: 20 per cent chose jobs classified as social class 3. Thus, in conclusion, the dynamic that determined high occupational aspirations among young black women appeared to be something other than the mothers' occupational status. It is to a further investigation of this question that I now turn: an investigation that examines the influence of *family* occupational background.

If we are adequately to gauge the social background of the young black women in the study who themselves are not yet in employment, and so cannot define their own social status, then we must assess as best we can the most representative social status of the family. Given that we are not in a position to redefine social classification schema[3], the most operative way to achieve this end would be to take the social class of the parent who could most adequately fulfil the head of household requirements laid down by conventional stratification theorists themselves. Goldthorpe (1983), articulating the conventional view, puts forward the following definition of the 'head of household'. He writes: 'The family "head" is the family member who has the greatest commitment to and continuity in the labour market' (p. 470). However, he then assumes: 'that this member is usually male is then an independent empirical observation' (p. 470).

It is my propostion here, contrary to conventional wisdom, that employed, married West Indian women in Britain can be defined as the 'head of household', and this is the important part, even when a husband is present. Furthermore I wish to argue that they can be defined as such by Goldthorpe's own criterion that states that the family head is the one who has the greatest commitment to and continuity in the labour market.

Goldthorpe regards any attempt to include married women into the class schema as 'problematic'. This he claims is because of the 'discontinuity so characteristic a feature of the employment histories of women' (p. 475). Goldthorpe makes the ethnocentric assumption that the majority of employed married women are working part-time and that their economic participation may have a somewhat impermanent and intermittent character as they enter or leave the labour force in response to the needs of child-care or the demands of a husband's career. However correct this may be for the majority of women in Britain (and that is questionable – see Beechey and Perkins 1987), it most certainly is not true for all and is particularly misleading with regard to the West Indian woman in Britain.

The evidence of this study, and indeed that of the PSI survey, *Black and White in Britain* (Brown 1984), suggests that there is no cultural precedent for making this ethnocentric assumption concerning West Indian women's commitment to the labour market. The characteristics of the black female workforce indicate that the social and economic contribution of the black woman to the British labour force is substantial. It is sufficient to merit recognition by any credible schema. Thus in the West Indian context to employ a convention that marginalises the female contribution and presumes that the male should be head of household when both partners equally contribute to the family would, in effect, distort social reality (Gill 1984; Massiah 1982, 1984, 1986, 1988).

Nancy Foner (1979), in her study of the West Indian migrant to Britain, makes an interesting observation. She presents evidence to suggest that to ignore the West Indian woman's occupational status in her own right would be problematic when trying to calculate occupational mobility. She shows that in fact the husbands of nearly all the white-collar and skilled women in her London sample were in jobs of a lower status than their wives, and many of them had experienced downward mobility in England. Thus, to consider the husband's occupational status and mobility experiences, rather than the woman's, would result in mis-classifying them as downwardly mobile instead of upwardly mobile.

In the same way it was apparent that not to take the females' occupational status into consideration when establishing the family background of the girls in the study would result in a misrepresentation. The families in my study would appear downwardly rather than upwardly skewed in the occupational hierarchy.[4] This was clearly illustrated by the figures which showed not only that the social class of the black male was much lower than that of the female, but the social class of the West Indian family to be substantially altered if the female was correctly incorporated into the schema.

In every respect the West Indian woman's labour-market commitment earns her the right to be recognised as capable of defining her family's social position. However, as already discussed, it is often the case that in determining parental background the conventional wisdom is to take the occupation of the male head of household. Studies of black occupational mobility persist in conforming to this methodological convention by maintaining that males are in every cultural setting still the most committed and involved in the labour market. It is this ethnocentric convention in established stratification analysis that has yet to be refuted successfully.

Returning to a consideration of the effect that family background has on occupational aspirations, we shall now consider data which show the relationship between the family social status and daughters' occupational aspirations. The social status of the West Indian families in the study is defined here in terms of occupation of that parent, either male or female, who most adequately fulfils the requirement of family head according to Goldthorpe's own definition. If both members appear to contribute equally to the family position then the parent with the higher social status was taken to be the definer of the family's social background.[5]

There appears to be a pattern in the data that indicates much the same trend that has been observed in our previous consideration of maternal and paternal occupational influence. The evidence suggests again that young black woman are choosing labour-market destinations independently of the occupational status of the head of household. This is shown by the fact that the majority of young women (over 70 per cent under any head of houshold grouping) chose careers in social class 1 and 2 (that is, professional and inter-mediate occupations). Girls from social class 3 families (namely, non-manual and manual) are as likely to choose occupations from their own social background as social class 1 and 2 girls, 20 per cent of whom wanted to do work classified as social class 3 occupations.

Other findings indicate that the majority of heads of households classified as professional and intermediate workers are in fact female (68 per cent). In the same way, male heads of household tend to be skilled manual workers (46 per cent). This finding, together with the observation that young black women aspire to high-status profes-sions, whether the heads of households are themselves manual or professional workers, presents further evidence that maternal or paternal social status is of little consequence in the decision-making process.

Among West Indians in Britain the link appears weak between the first and the second generation with regard to their occupational aspirations. This suggests that young black women do not necessarily wish to reproduce their social-class status, however defined. The question then arises as to how the West Indian parent influences his or her child.

RE-EVALUATING PARENTAL INFLUENCE

In this study there appeared to be two ways in which parents influenced aspirations: one, the positive orientation to education, and the other, the black female orientation to work, both of which can be regarded as British West Indian working-class characteristics. I shall now turn to an assessment of these two important class characteristics in order that we may move towards some explanation for the high aspirations of young black women.

1 First- and second-generation attitudes to education

It is often the case that people migrate for 'a better life'. This is as true of the West Indians who came to the UK as any other group of people. West Indians came to Britain in the 1950s, in what can be argued as *both* a male- and female-headed migration, in search of better opportunities for themselves and their children. While objectively occupational opportunities for migrants are restricted by specific constraints with regard to their disadvantaged labour-market position, there is another dimension to migrant life: that of their own subjective occupational orientation.

This internal cultural dynamic of migrants, what I call the 'migrant effect', refers to the degree to which migrants themselves pursue the goal of upward occupational mobility, particularly for the next generation, by striving for educational achievement and qualifications. The influence of this 'migrant effect' on educational outcomes may vary according to the culture of the migrant group, the country of settlement, and economic and social conditions (especially significant is the extent of racial exclusion and discrimination), but it nevertheless remains a characteristic feature among many migrant groups (Alba 1985).

Glazer and Moynihan (1963) discuss in *Beyond the Melting Pot*, their study of American migrant society, the drive for educational credentials among the many migrant groups in the USA. They describe the Jews' 'passion' for education; the Italian concept of (family) social status through the professional occupations of their children; the Puerto Rican capacity for hard work and the value they place on schooling. Of the West Indian migrants who came to the USA in 1920–1925 Glazer and Moynihan write: 'The ethos of the West Indians . . . emphasised saving, hard work, investment and education . . . buying homes and in general advancing themselves' (p. 35).

They remark that West Indians, such as Marcus Garvey, 'furious' at the prejudice they encountered in America (which they felt was far greater than that among the whites in their home islands), turned to radical politics.

Leggett (in Bettelheim and Janowitz 1977) supports this thesis of political involvement, claiming that blacks, having the lowest ethnic status have therefore the highest level of class consciousness. Indeed, a degree of political consciousness among early black migrants to the UK has been demonstrated by the 'Black Education movement' set up by this generation of migrants (Chevannes 1979; Tomlinson 1985). The struggle for basic educational rights has been a political focal point for the 'black community' since the 1960s. However, as Tomlinson observes, it is not so much a radical movement as one that seeks to ensure equality of opportunity for migrant children within the education system. Confirming that migrant parents have strong educational aspirations for their children, Tomlinson (1982) writes:

The parents very much aware of the discrimination their children could face in seeking employment after school placed great faith in the acquisition of educational qualifications to help overcome this.

(p. 34)

Parental recognition that the British education system discriminates against the black child has resulted in the establishment of black supplementary schools, spearheaded by the action, in particular, of black women. These separate black schools embody the belief that education will ultimately help black children to succeed in an 'English' system by providing them with the credentials necessary for employment, or further education and training in the majority society.

It was found in the study that black parents wanted improved educational standards for their children, and despite the general feeling of disillusionment and mistrust towards the schools their daughters attended, still retained their faith in the meritocratic ideal. Among the parents interviewed it was clear that securing educational opportunities for their children was of central importance, as one father explained:

We work to give our children opportunity. We earn to pay rent, buy a little food. Man, there was no time for bettering ourself. Our children, they now have the benefits to better theyself, education and so on. We didn't have these opportunities, our childrens now have these opportunities and we's work hard for them. [sic]

(Mr Burgess, London Regional Transport maintenance)

Parents were 'realistic' about employment opportunities, and their knowledge of British racism, gained from their own experience, made them anxious for their children. They had a clear understanding of the 'make-or-break' situation that faced their children in Britain today, as Mrs Pierre, a mother of one of the girls, explained:

When we came here, there was so many jobs, we could've move from one to another. The first night I arrive I get a job with my cousin. But the more of us come the less work, but we had relatives then an' that make it easier. But now these children, they don't understand. They have it harder to get a job now, there is much against them that we not have then. But now they have opportunity. We are here to help them get on and we can help them educate themselves. They don't have to find the money for rent. You see, we had our children here and so they grow up expecting different things.

> (Mrs Pierre: auxiliary night nurse)

Clark (1983) puts forward a theory as to why poor black families succeed in education. He argues that too often studies emphasise family composition (that is, single-parent families or others) and not family disposition (beliefs and values). This is an important point; black girls in the study did seem to derive much of their determination for 'getting on' from their parental orientation and both the passive and active support this engendered. It was apparent that West Indian parents did encourage their daughters and were proud of their successes in many different ways. A parent, a canteen worker for 24 years since her arrival from Jamaica in 1954, outlined her ideas and values on education and her daughters' success:

> It is important that she does what she wants, then she will do well. . . . Anita should stay on and finish her studies. I does see many that leave, hang around the streets, what is the point of leaving school to do this? Our other daughter, Sheila, she went to John Henry school, did well and then went on to college, then a Government job. They send her on a social work training course, CQSW I think it called. She probably out working today, she's a residential social worker now. The next one she does something with computers. Me, I don't understand a thing about that. My's only fear is Anita, now she start saying she want to be a nun. It's that school, you know. What will she do when we want to play we music, drink and relax? [sic]

Parental attitudes to their children's education varied from those who took strong disciplinarian measures to those who adopted a passive approach. The passive approach was an attitude that relied heavily on trust between parent and child, and much responsibility lay with the child. Ms Dean, a cleaner in a West End hotel, describes what was the passive support role of many parents in the study:

> She's a good girl, goes up and works on her own. Some children at school disturb her. Some children want to work, others don't. You know there are just some children like that. We never force them to work, there is no point, it must come from themselves.

This type of parental support was often misunderstood by the school. Teachers argued that this form of parental concern was not sufficient for the girls' needs, and often complained that it led to over-ambitiousness among the pupils. For example, Ms Parker, a fifth-form mistress, had this to say of one parent who was an educational welfare officer: 'The problem is that she believes you must work hard to get anywhere, to move out of your circumstances, this philosophy has got through to Sherry who is just too over-ambitious for her ability.'

It was clear that teachers, rather than considering it an asset, considered passive parental encouragement to be negative, as the following comment made by a teacher concerning a black parent shows:

> The mother wants too much of her daughter, she is far too over-ambitious for her. Just to show you she really hasn't a clue about her daughter, she's only capable of a low-grade CSE and she wants her to do 'O' levels.

Another teacher had this to say of the passive, but supportive, role of one family: 'The parents are not unduly worried as she works hard but she is just not able enough to carry it off, she is not geared up to the exam level.'

The evidence showed that in many cases black parents attempted to provide whatever support they were able to give, mostly of a moral and where possible a material nature. It was clear that many working-class black parents, not least because of their own educational background or the restrictions induced by difficult working conditions, rely heavily on the school to provide the less accessible material and academic help they were often unable to give.

Nevertheless, it must be noted that however 'conservative' the parental attitudes towards education appeared to be, this acceptance of the status quo was not reflected in the cultural ideology of the West Indian working class. They often referred to the racism they knew existed in society and in the classroom. The setting up of supplementary schools, with its emphasis on high educational standards, bears witness to this fact. The apparent contradiction between the desire for a traditional education and the need for radical politics did not appear to be problematic to the West Indian working-class community, who found it a logical stance in the light of their migrant experience and the racism they had encountered. Ms Arnold rationalises these seemingly opposite views in the following passage:

I does get real angry when they say the Queen's prejudice, she invited us here. I remember the day my friend brought a Gazette and showed me the headline, 'Immigrants Welcome, Queen Welcomes Immigrants'. We was sitting under a tree in the shade, that's when I make up me mind to come. She invited us here, how can they be prejudiced if they ask us to come? She is Head of State in the West Indies. The problem is they don't know their history here, these English people. [sic]

However, Mrs Arnold went on to explain the reality of life and bringing up children in this country and in so doing presented a different ideological position:

It's bad, real bad. . . . The school has a lot of it [racism]. I know because it was real difficult to get Verne in the school . . . there are so few blacks there and you know the reason why. I know the teachers are racist, but you must be careful because they are the teachers and until you leave that is a problem. Them can be vengeful and harm your child's prospects, this is a real racist place. [sic]

Parents were also aware of the problems faced by black youth but did not associate the difficulties they encountered with the police with anything other than racism and state coercion. Despite their disciplinarian values, which often prompted them to complain of the laziness of young people, parents were aware of the political issues involved. Mrs Davis talked about the bad media publicity blacks get and the level of police harassment which they encounter:

I tell you there's no wonder there so much trouble. They [the police] really ask for it the way they treat us black people. But the way the papers report it you'll never know what really go on, you see. In Brixton I was in the middle of it. The things I saw . . . pushing two black boys into a van, then they just start kicking and beating upon them on the floor. A next boy he run up to help but they just turn on him too. Man, I just turn and ran. (Daughter, listening, says, 'I hate them.')

Nancy Foner (1979), in the late 1970s, made the following observation about the likely orientation of West Indian migrants' children towards education in the years to come. She wrote:

The struggle to get a good education may, however, become a central focus in their lives; the second generation set their goals higher than their parents have and measure their achievements and prospects by English rather than Jamaican standards.

(p. 217)

Indeed, as Foner predicted, the second-generation West Indian girls in the study did show a strong commitment to education and in particular identified with the meritocratic ideal as a means of 'getting on'. This was clearly illustrated in the girls' optimistic statements:

Black people work hard and want to really make something of themselves. I want to get on in my life.
(Marsha: aspiration, social work; mother: office worker; father: carpenter)

I believe you can really change things for yourself, it is up to you but you really can.
(Laurie: aspiration, journalist; mother: secretary; father: telephonist)

The strategy of 'staying on' in pursuit of educational qualifications was the way many working-class black women expressed their aspirations for 'getting on' in life, as the following extracts show:

My plans are to stay in education until I get my 'A' levels. Then I plan to go to college to become a social worker.
(Sherry; mother: social worker; father: BR engineer; ability high)

I want to stay on and then go to college so that I might study journalism.
(Veronica; mother: cook; father: mechanic; ability average)

While West Indian working-class parental attitudes were an important factor in motivating the girls, there was substantial evidence that the specific choice of career was greatly influenced by a realistic self-appraisal of their academic capabilities. Girls did not aspire to careers that they felt they would not be able to achieve whatever the parental occupational status, as a comparison between the following statements show:

I would like to do medicine especially something to do with women and the curing of disease.
(Isabel; mother: midwife; father: labourer; ability high)

I would like to be a legal secretary and work in an office.
(Joy; mother: insurance officer; father: accountant; ability low)

If I leave school I would go to college and do a BEC general course, after that I would do a BEC national and then HND so then I have got a wide range of jobs which I will be able to do.

(Selma; mother: nurse; father: telephone engineer; ability average)

I would like to study and learn about computers. I'd like to do data processing as it is something interesting and that I will be able to do.

(Sharon; mother: cleaner; father: absent; ability average)

It was notable, however, that the higher the social status of the parent the more likely it was that the daughter would choose to go on into higher education, rather than further education, as a means of qualifying for a profession. Two statements, set against the context of their parental status, illustrated this process of exclusion:

I would like to go on and do a degree in psychology, preferably at a polytechnic.

(Jackie; mother: cook; father: welder; ability high)

I would like to do a BA degree in business studies, in accounts and then study for a chartered accountant degree at university.

(Floya; mother: playgroup leader; father: chartered accountant; ability high)

In this way social class can be seen to have some effect on the accessibility of higher education. However, as Tomlinson (1983b) in her study on black women in higher education shows, many of the young women at university were from working-class social backgrounds. Indeed, the aspiration towards a university education was not exclusive to girls of professional parents, and several young black women from working-class backgrounds did indicate that they would like to go on to university:

I would like to stay on at school and do three 'A' levels. After I would like to get into a university and get a degree in law. I intend to be a barrister and practise law.

(Ruby; mother: nursery teacher; father: clerk; ability high)

I want to do a degree course somewhere that I know.

(Frances; mother: social worker; father: postman; ability high)

Their coming from single-parent backgrounds did not necessarily limit the girls' aspirations, especially if their ability was high:

I have already got six 'O' levels. Now I am doing three more and some 'A' levels so that I can study interior design. I want to go to the London School of Furniture.

(Debra; mother: local government officer; father: absent (postman); ability high)

I would like, finally, to do art therapy, after doing a course at Goldsmiths' [University of London].

(Avril; mother deceased; father: painter-decorator; ability high)

Nonetheless, the goal of higher education among black working-class girls of high ability was the exception rather than the rule. It was notable that the majority of young black women did aspire to Further Education college whatever their ability, most of them seeking work in a social/caring profession.

An explanation for high black female aspirations has been attempted by Fuller (1982). While she was right to observe the girls' commitment and resoluteness in their efforts to achieve their goals, she was less correct in describing this positive orientation as a 'subculture of resistance', the outcome of a reaction to negative parental and societal pressures towards black females. The explanation for their positive orientation seemed to lie within an understanding of the transmission of the West Indian migrant, working-class ethos, the values of which had filtered down to the girls from their parents, and had subsequently been modified.[6] Many of the young women in the study described how their parents had an important role to play not only in influencing their cultural identity, but also in shaping their specific educational outlooks, both of which combined to make them what they were today:

Both my parents brought me up in the West Indian way. They brought me and are still bringing me up in the way their parents brought them up. I would like to pass this West Indian tradition down to my children so that this tradition lives on and never dies.

(Karen; mother: nurse; father: London Regional Transport maintenance)

As we grew up my parents used to talk about 'back home' and how it differed from England. Although I was born in England I always felt attached to my parents' country. . . . If our parents did not pass down some of their culture black people would lose out on a lot of things, e.g. who their ansister [sic] was, and how they lived and how they differed from white people and their culture.

(Merle; mother: cleaner; father: bus conductor)

The Church was also an important part of West Indian working-class life, and it was not uncommon to find the girls expressing a religious influence in their career decision.[7] One girl stated: 'I would like to be a successful business woman with God's help, it gives me strength to know He guides me' (Janet; mother: teacher; father: carpenter). Several other girls who stated that God was a major source of encouragement also taught at Sunday school at the weekend.

Being second-generation West Indian meant that, unlike their parents, these young women also saw themselves as British. Having a black British identity was not considered problematic.[8] The girls had few illusions about being accepted as being British, and maintained a second-generation modified form of 'West Indianness' among them, as the following statements reveal:

I may have been born here but I do not feel that I am English, simply because I have not been given the chance to feel English. I do feel that I am black though, but that I live in England.

(Karen; mother: nurse; father: London Regional Transport
maintenance)

I am me because my parents have taught me a lot of their ways, and being brought up in a British society has combined to make me what I am today.

(Julie; mother: cook; father: absent)

I have only ever lived in England, but my parents are Dominican. I think England is a nice country but the people are false. Because one minute they are talking to you and the next they are talking behind your back, which is not very nice. In England there are a lot of prejudices which you do not find in other countries. So even though I have a British passport I don't only class myself as British but as Dominican too.

(Denise; mother: cook; father: unemployed)

The girls were aware of managing the separate spheres of school and home life. In the following extract of a classroom conversation, the teacher asks the black girls in the class about the problems of a 'generation gap':

Ms James: But do you not find there to be different aspirations between you and your parents?

Dianne: You get used to it.

Merle: You don't do it at home, you'll get told off, but you do it at school, you don't bother.

The strong emphasis on discipline and doing 'what was expected of you' in the West Indian household was acknowledged by the girls to be part of their culture and ultimately practised by their parents in their best interests.

My mother came here to get a better education for her children, sometimes if you feel you don't want to go to school . . . well, you just have to feel you want to.

(Dianne; mother: dinner lady; father: ticket collector)

Back home it's stricter there, beating and all that. Sometimes it's not good. They expect too much of you for your age. Beat you if you don't pass a test and all that, but I tell you it makes you work!

(Ann; mother: nurse; father: plumber)

My parents brought me up very well, a little bit restricted but it doesn't bother me.

(Dawn; mother: cook; father: unemployed)

It was found that the girls held similar expectations about discipline and control to those of their parents. This accounted for their often stated preference for strong discipline in the classroom, which they identified as 'control', and organised, structured lessons which they regarded as 'good teaching'. In the girls' statements it was clear what they considered a good education to be:

Since I have been here things have got so bad. Miss Grey [the headmistress] has got no control, things are out of hand, I would say.

(Kara: upper-sixth-form student)

There is no discipline downstairs [i.e., lower school] . . . it's disgusting.

(Frances: upper-sixth-form student)

As a consequence of their educational expectations, it was not uncommon to find that girls were often disillusioned with the type of teaching they were receiving. It was clear that the young women had developed a strategy by which they gauged those lessons and teachers that were worth listening to. The girls were obviously bored and uninterested in the 'liberal teaching' approach of some teachers. In these often relaxed and less structured classes the girls would sit in the back of the room and carry on with 'prep', neither being disruptive nor participating.

This was also the case with teachers whom the girls judged to be indifferent or uncaring and with lessons they considered a waste of time.[9] Fuller (1982) suggests that the negative classroom stance which she also observed among the girls in her study was a manifestation of the 'subcultural' resistance to authority prevalent among alienated black females. However, there was little evidence to support this view of their often obvious classroom dissent. The girls appeared to be getting on with their own work as a means of rationalising what they considered to be unproductive and wasteful lesson time. Their response to certain (though not all)[10] teachers was the outcome of the girls' particular and unique orientation to education, which was clearly the product of their West Indian social class background.

2 The black female working-class orientation to work

Women are socialised to be resourceful. Each succeeding generation learns from the preceding one what it takes to survive in an environment often unfavorable to women.

(Justus 1985:447)

While there appeared to be no direct association between the maternal social-class occupational status and daughters' aspirations, data from other sources indicated that the second-generation girls were greatly influenced by their mothers' work experience. The way in which the previous female migrant generation affected their daughters' orientation to work was clearly illustrated in the statements and decisions made by young black women. Within the context of a cultural consideration of social class, a unique female work tradition is revealed which clearly has an important influence on the aspirations of succeeding generations.

If we begin with an investigation into the characteristics of this unique black female work tradition, the distinctive nature of their experience vis-à-vis their white working-class counterparts becomes evident. In the study, 84 per cent of the black mothers worked, 69 per cent in full-time employment. This contrasted sharply with the other mothers in the study, of whom only 46 per cent worked, 28 per cent full-time. White women were also almost twice as likely to be unpaid workers (29 per cent) – a type of work often referred to as housework – than black women (13 per cent).

Despite the limited scale of this investigation this was by no means an unrepresentative sample. The PSI (Brown 1984) statistics and the Labour Force Survey (OPCS 1987) revealed similar trends in the national population. For example, PSI stated that 74 per cent of black women in the UK worked, and of these women only 29 per cent were in part-time employment. In the indigenous population, 46 per cent of the women worked and most of these were in part-time employment (46 per cent).

The black female cohort differed from the white women in the sample in other ways too, in that black women were more likely to head their households. Both in terms of the traditional definition of a female-headed household (that is, one where a husband is not present); and according to the more equitable definition (the most economically committed and better situated in the occupational hierarchy). This study showed that 45 per cent of West Indian women headed their household compared to 11 per cent of white women.

Sutton and Makiesky-Barrow (1977), in their study of Barbadian society, make this comment about the West Indian female orientation to work:

> Women are expected not only to contribute to their own and their children's support but also to acquire and build separate economic resources, control their own earnings and use them as they see fit. Men readily accept the idea of their wives working; in fact a man might boast of his wife's position and earnings.
>
> (p. 307)

Clearly the evidence does suggest that West Indian women do have different relationships within their families and, in particular, with the males in these families, that contribute to a unique working tradition. Barrow (1986) suggests that men and relationships with men were an important part of enhancing female economic autonomy and were not a restriction in the traditional Euro-centred sense; nor, as some authors suggest (Wilson 1969), only a means of gaining social respectability. Explanations as to why this may be so point to the central concept of an ideology of meritocracy in West Indian workingclass life, in which both men and women appear to participate equally (Jules 1991). As Sutton and Makiesky-Barrow (1977) observe:

The position a woman acquires often results from her own achievements rather than her spouse and women tend to be individually ranked even if they are married. Although both sexes speak critically of status ranking and its negative role in the social life of the community, status mobility is in fact a major concern. Women as well as men are preoccupied with finding a way of 'rising' a notch above within the social hierarchy, and both look to the occupational system for doing so.

(p. 302)

Lee (1982) makes the following interesting observation with regard to the ideology of meritocracy and its effects on the equality of opportunity between the sexes. He writes with regard to the Irish situation:

The less a culture emphasises merit, the more resistant to equality are the males likely to be . . . if only because the supremacy of the dominant males does not depend on superior merit. They are therefore likely to feel vulnerable to what they perceive as a threat posed not so much by women, as by ability in women.

(p. 10)

In a culture that places a value on merit, such as the West Indian working-class culture in Britain, this syndrome that Lee describes in the Irish situation does not appear to arise in the black British context. It would seem from the evidence given by the males in the study that female labour-market participation is not perceived as a threat to their own economic and social status.

Barrow (1986) also moves some way towards accounting for the characteristically positive labour-market orientation and tradition of economic independence evident among working-class West Indian women in the Caribbean. She argues that the struggle for economic autonomy was a necessary strategy for survival, a form of self-reliance should other forms of economic support fail, or be insufficient to meet their often most basic requirements. Barrow makes the important observation that the black women's rationale for working was not about gaining social mobility, nor even escaping from poverty, but rather a means to 'achieve mere survival and mark time with occasional improvements in standards of living' (p. 170). It could be argued that this strategy, evident among the migrant generation, has been passed down and modified by the second generation, who themselves, seeking a modicum of upward mobility, still appear to employ a similar rationale.

In the interview data provided by the young black women, strong feelings about the need to work were evident (see Chapter 6). In their expression of this desire, these women located the essential role of their mothers (or female guardian or relative) as an important inspir- ation, as the following statements show:

I want to be like my mother, well liked, sociable, outgoing and most of all successful.

> (Joanna; aspiration: teacher; mother: secretary)

Both my mother and sister do book-keeping and accounts. I would like to follow in their footsteps and do as well in my job as they have done in theirs.

> (Trudi; aspiration: office work; mother: book-keeper)

My mother has had to work hard to bring us up, and she brings us up in the West Indian ways. She's had to take shit at work, but I think she's brave.

> (Anita; aspiration: social work; mother: cook)

In response to the question 'Who do you admire most?', a total of 20 per cent of young black women positively indicated their mother, other female relative (such as grandmother, aunt or sister) or female friend. This was in contrast to their white female peers of whom only 8 per cent said that they were influenced by any female associate, whether mother or sister.

When asked if they would like to do the same type of work as their mothers, however, the girls nearly always replied 'No'. It was clear, therefore, that it was not the mothers' actual job that influ- enced the girls as much as their mothers' (and other black females') attitudes and rational strategies. This aspect of occupational influence can be seen if a comparison is made between actual maternal occu- pation and daughters' aspirations.

For example, while 20 per cent of black girls' mothers were employed as nurses, only half as many of their daughters wished to pursue such a career (10 per cent). In fact, when asked what job did they most dislike, 32 per cent of the young black women indicated that nursing was the job they would like the least, suggesting that a reason for the decision was the type of work and that they knew of women, often their mothers, who did it.

Although a large number of mothers were engaged in unskilled and semi-skilled 'caring' and 'service' work (for example, 27 per cent of the mothers were employed as home-helps, dinner ladies and cleaners), virtually none of their daughters showed any inclination to undertake such work. The only work that they desired to do that was classified as unskilled and semi-skilled was associated with child-care. Another popular choice being made by the girls that did not reflect their mothers' labour-market experience was their desire to do office work. Whereas 20 per cent stated their desire to do such work, only 10 per cent of their mothers had been successful in securing such jobs.

On the whole the careers being selected by the girls reflected a much broader range of jobs than those in which their mothers were currently employed. Jobs in journalism, artistic careers of various sorts, jobs in business and the medical and academic professions, were some of the careers chosen by the girls of which their mothers had little experience.

CONCLUSION: THE CULTURAL CONTEXT OF SOCIAL CLASS

A conventional examination of the influence of social class, examining paternal, maternal and heads of households' occupational status on young black women's career choices demonstrated that by this method no association could be found. Young black women, whatever the occupational status of their parents, maintained, in general, high aspirations of social class.

However, a detailed consideration of West Indian working-class, migrant cultural characteristics revealed that, in fact, young black women were strongly influenced by their parents' orientation to work and education. It could be argued positive attitudes to education and the lack of restrictions on female labour market participation within West Indian families account for the high aspirations of social class amongst these girls. The case for a cultural reappraisal of social class therefore appeared valid in view of this evidence.

Chapter 9

Conclusion

Understanding inequality

We are all brought up in the belief that, no matter who you are, if you work hard and do well at school you will be rewarded in the world of work. This is the 'meritocratic ideal': a fundamental pillar of liberal democratic society.

It is an ideal enshrined within the British educational system. The goal of 'equality of opportunity' that it embraces suggests that the occupational outcomes of pupils should be a reflection of their educational achievements regardless of class, race or gender. If this is so, how then do we account for those who do well at school yet still fail to rise up the occupational ladder? This study, which examined the career aspirations and expectations of second-generation African Caribbean young women up to and at the point of their entry into the labour market, addressed this question.

Young black women bear all the hallmarks of a fundamentally inegalitarian society. They do well at school, contribute to society, are good, efficient workers yet, as a group, they consistently fail to secure the economic status and occupational prestige they deserve. This study asked why it is that black women suffer these injustices, and attempted to reveal the processes of inequality, that, despite the ideology of a meritocracy, persist in this society.

The findings of this study showed that the career choices being made by these second-generation African Caribbean women were, relative to their peers, both high and distinct. In terms of social class the majority of young black women both expected and aspired to jobs in the highest social grouping. Of young black women 74 per cent indicated that they both expected and aspired to get jobs in social class 1 and 2. These jobs, often (though not always) identifiable as traditional female 'professional and intermediate' occupations, were located particularly in the social and welfare 'caring' fields. Of the 20 per cent who aspired to jobs classified in social class 3, 10 per cent indicated their preference for non-manual, mainly office-type, work, while 10 per cent stated their preference for skilled manual employment, again largely of the 'caring' variety.

In contrast, young black men, though also aspiring to higher social-class occupations than white male peers (but lower than those of their black female counterparts), were less likely to expect to achieve their aspirations in the job market. On the whole they expected to find employment as skilled manual workers.

Compared to their black female peers, young white women were more likely to aspire to and expect to secure employment in social class 3, as non-manual and skilled manual workers. Young white men were the least likely of any of the pupils to want or expect a job in social class 1 and 2. Their preference for skilled manual work was marked. However, a fair proportion of young white men did aspire and expect to be employed as non-manual workers, which was in sharp contrast to the young black men, none of whom indicated that they thought this area of employment was accessible to them.

In attempting to account for the distinct aspirations of the young black women, the influence of social class on the cohort was examined. The findings suggested that, contrary to those studies which assert that there is little or no social class influence on West Indian occupational choice (Sillitoe and Meltzer 1985), there was in fact a clear association. This association, however, was not immediately apparent in a conventional examination of maternal, paternal or parental social class. Young black women, whatever the occupational status of their parents, maintained high social-class aspirations.

A detailed consideration of working-class West Indian migrant cultural characteristics suggested that second-generation West Indian migrant women were influenced by their parents' orientation to work and education. Positive attitudes towards education and the lack of constraint on female labour-market participation within West Indian families, it was found, accounted in part for young black women's high social-class aspirations.

The nature of the West Indian female orientation to the labour market formed a central argument in the book. In response to the dominant and established explanations for black female motivation – that is, the strong role model of the mother figure and in the particular their 'unique' orientation to motherhood (Driver 1980b; Fuller 1982; Phizacklea 1982; Dex 1983; Eggleston et al. 1986) – it was found that the young black women in the study expressed what was essentially an ideology emphasising the relative autonomy of both the male and female roles. Like their parents and grandparents, these young black women had not adopted the dominant Euro-centric ideology: an ideology in which gender was regarded as the basis for the opposition of roles and values.

The evidence suggested that the cultural construction of femininity among African Caribbean women fundamentally differed from forms of femininity found among their white peers, especially their white migrant (Irish) peers. In the black definition, the statements revealed that few distinctions were made between male and female abilities and attributes with regard to work and the labour market. This particular definition of masculinity and femininity resulted in greater female participation because nothing in the definitions of appropriate sex-role behaviour excluded them from areas of social and economic achievement.

The factors so far described account for the commitment to a full-time career and the presence of high social-class aspirations evident among young black women, but the marked tendency to opt for careers in what are commonly classified as traditional female occupational preserves also needed to be explained.

It was found that the usual processes held to structure gender disadvantage in this society are further complicated by both the operation of racism and the distinct ideological orientation of working-class African Caribbean young women. Clearly what these girls were doing was attempting to achieve some measure of upward occupational mobility by means of a strategy that rationalised in their interests the various educational and labour-market constraints that they encountered.

A major constraint was the existence of a racially and sexually segregated labour market which ensured limited occupational opportunities open to young black women. The black girls chose jobs that were 'gendered', such as social work, nursing or office work, not so much because of the nature of the job, but because that was the only type of work in their experience and knowledge that was available to them. However, in choosing these jobs, they used the stated educational requirements as a vehicle for obtaining more or better qualifications, in an effort to enhance their career prospects and satisfy their desire for credentials. Their willingness to move into 'non-gendered' careers (relative to their white peers) can largely be explained by the combination of the notion of relative equality between the sexes, which ensured that there were no cultural limits to their attempts to do non-traditional, female work, and the motivation to succeed, which encouraged the search for all available opportunities.

A crucial factor in shaping the distinct occupational aspirations of young black women was the experience of schooling. As a vital resource to black female pupils who were about to enter the labour market, schools were seen to play an important role in both structuring and restricting black female occupational aspirations and expectations. Confirming the findings of the Eggleston Report (Eggleston *et al*. 1986), it was found, that with regard to information, advice and educational preparation, schools often failed their black pupils.

Black girls were clearly not being provided with the appropriate levels of qualifications needed to enter the labour market in accordance with their ability. A comparative evaluation of the two schools in the study supported the findings of the ILEA study conducted by Peter Mortimore (Mortimore *et al*. 1988), suggesting that the school which an individual pupil attended did make a difference. As an investigation of their examination results showed, black girls fared poorly within the 'selective' grammar school ethos of St Theresa's. Here, lower-ability girls, many of whom were black, experienced (not least because of the system of recruitment) five years of what effectively was seen to be 'custodial' education. St Hilda's, with its record of academic 'mediocrity' and poor standards of teaching, meant that all, but in particular the bright black girls, did not do as well as they could have done in their examinations.

Furthermore, it was observed that much of the girls' time at school was spent using strategies to avoid the effects of racist and negative teacher expectations. Strategies such as not taking up a specific subject or not asking for help were employed as the only means of challenging their teachers' expectations of them; expectations that were often characterised by the practice of either overt or unintentional racism.

Black girls were not only impeded by teachers' assessments of their abilities, but their decision making was fundamentally influenced by the poverty of advice and information they received about job opportunities. Primarily because they were not given the opportunity to explore other possibilities, young black women often chose their careers from a limited range of occupations, depending on their own knowledge and existing experience of the labour market. In this respect both the Careers Education Programme and the Careers

Service were found wanting. Confused in their role, poorly resourced and underdeveloped, they provided little direction to those who relied most heavily on their services.

The quality of other aspects of vocational preparation in the schools was also questionable. In a similar finding to Austin (1987), recruitment to YTS from the schools was seen to be clearly discriminatory, with low-level schemes being aimed at those who were thought of as unemployable. The demand for early subject specialisation in the third year was not complemented by adequate guidance, nor was it free of teacher prejudice. Information in the upper school, especially the sixth form, was inappropriate for the needs of the black girls who stayed on to re-sit vital exams or wished to go on into further and higher education.

Diego Gambetta (1988), in a study about the educational decision-making process, interestingly entitled *Were They Pushed or Did They Jump?*, suggests that individuals tend to evaluate rationally the conditions under which they make educational decisions according to the cost and benefits of their choices. He concludes that people subject to economic constraints adjust their expectations according to their own academic ability and their labour-market benefits, suggesting that if anything individuals jump rather than are pushed.

Young black women did make rational choices based on ability and job opportunity, but in the context of overwhelming institutional limitations, and under the severe economic constraints of a racially and sexually determined labour market. In these conditions the issue of rational choice, as discussed by Gambetta, becomes somewhat academic. The women in the study found themselves in a position where, in order to achieve a modicum of upward mobility, they had little choice but to turn the limited educational and labour-market opportunities open to them to their advantage.

Educational research that addresses the issue of race in schools has shown little commitment to an investigation of gender (Mirza 1986a). As the Swann Report (DES 1985) exemplifies, the possibility of acknowledging black achievement seems problematic to those wishing to assert simplistic models of race, culture and underachievement. To those writing about the issue of race in the labour market, a similar tendency to marginalise the findings on women as 'uncharacteristic' or 'spurious' prevails.

The presence of high aspirations in the context of continuing labour-market inequality acts as a clear indictment of the failure of a meritocratic ideology to provide a more egalitarian society. As Halsey, Heath and Ridge (1980) have argued, it was the hope of the architects of the 1944 Education Act, and later those who campaigned for the 1976 move towards comprehensivisation, that a more equitable educational system could be achieved. But the occupational outcomes of the young black women in the study, four years after leaving school, were clearly not a reflection of their educational potential or achievements.

In conclusion, the evidence presented in this book suggested that ultimately, whatever the educational level or labour-market disposition of these young black women, their occupational location was subject to a variety of factors; in particular, labour market structures and educational resources. Inequalities based on race, gender and class remain an integral feature of this society in spite of its ideology of meritocracy.

RECOMMENDATIONS

Burney's (1988) findings with regard to the limited effect of existing equal opportunities legislation (including the temporary effect of any 'package' of positive discrimination), together with the rather pessimistic conclusions of this research project, suggest that any policy recommendations aimed at redressing inequality may be little more than cosmetic. However, the investigations of this study do point to two important policy *directions*.

1 A reappraisal of social policy and the black family

In his study of the black condition in America, Wilson (1987) suggests that public policy initiatives aimed at stemming the tide of the growing black 'underclass' should be directed at restoring the economically successful, self-assured, black male breadwinner. The persistent attack on the black family, and in particular the identification of the single mother as a major cause of black disadvantage, is a continuing misrepresentation in social policy, arising from the reluctance to acknowledge anything other than the nuclear conjugal family as the norm.

The findings of this study suggest that young black women have an alternative and equally valid concept of the family. Based on the notion of relative autonomy between the sexes, relationships and parenthood are determined by compatibility between partners and not the promise of economic security within the institution of marriage. That this pattern has endured historically, and in times of economic hardship increases, is evidence of its viability and value.

The single-parent unit, rather than being an indicator of 'low cultural morality', the emasculation of the black male and the weakened black family (Moynihan 1965, in Rainwater and Yancey 1967; Murray 1984:1990), appears to be a positive and strategic life-style (Phoenix 1990). However, the lack of recognition that motherhood solicits, in terms of social policy and institutional resources in Britain, compared to any other western nation is well documented (Moss and Brannen 1988; McRobbie 1990).

Although the facilitation of women in their careers as mothers and workers receives a great deal of lip-service from the government, it receives little financial investment. This shallow commitment towards child-care is yet again firm evidence of the decreasing social concern of the government, who seem to have as a central goal of their employment policy a determination to discourage women from participating in any sphere other than the domestic.

Vital support services, such as state provision for the under-fives, nurseries, day-care, work-place crèches, after-school care; other basic rights, such as child-care and maternity allowances, maternity leave; and important employment concessions, such as job-share and part-time hours – all have in real terms been either eroded or ignored by a government that is prepared to leave child-care and education to the determinants of the (male) market-place (EOC 1990). However, it is precisely these services, and the recognition of better pay for women's work, that all black women, who are now an integral part of the British economy (see Westwood and Bhachu 1988) require in order that they can secure better standards of living for themselves and their children.

2 'Magnetising the masses'

The findings of this research project clearly showed the problems faced by inner-city schools and the effect this had on the black pupils within them. The need for better career-information services, better standards of teaching and leadership, better resources and facilities and, in particular, a more effective anti-racist strategy (as indicated by the Burnage Report, Runnymede Trust 1989; see also Sivanandan 1990, Gilroy 1990, and Shah 1990) are required to raise the level of schooling that black pupils receive. Black parents, teachers and pupils have long demanded such basic rights (see Stone 1985; Chevannes and Reeves 1987; Shah 1989).

In a statement Neil Fletcher, who was at the time the leader of the now defunct radical ILEA (Inner London Education Authority), describes such a policy that would raise the standards of pupils of *all* inner city schools as 'a Mark II comprehensive model' (*Guardian*, 13 October 1987). Based on the American notion of 'magnet schools', set up to serve bright black ghetto children, Fletcher calls for a 'magnetising of the masses'. This, he suggests, is attainable by increasing working-class parental participation, establishing 'quality control' by means of proper attainment tests, increasing incentives for classroom and head-teachers, and monitoring the size and ability intake of pupils into any one school.

However, the move to improve standards has not originated from this quarter, but has come instead in the form of the enforced and haphazard requirements of Kenneth Baker's 1988 Education Reform Act which came into effect in 1990 (David 1989; Flude and Hammer 1989; Troyna 1990). With its politically inspired changes for 'opting out', a national curriculum, and greater centralisation (see 1991 Schools Charter, *Independent*, 5 June 1991), the Act has all the hallmarks of what Ainley (1988) has described as 'a new Victorian era in education'. Far from raising standards, through the medium of 'parental choice', and instilling academic rigour into the lives of our children, it will in effect reinstate a system of selectivity, which instead of 'magnetising the masses' will ride roughshod over all the progress of the recent decades, re-establishing instead large pockets of inequality within the educational system.

Notes

2 The myth of underachievement

1 Even research investigating scholastic success suggested that it was the children of middle-class black parents who would do well at school, unlike their working-class counterparts (Bagley, Bart and Wong 1979).

2 The study of race relations in America is focused around the ongoing and controversial debate concerning the structure and development of the black family. See Ryan 1971; Gutman 1976; Jones 1986; Wilson 1987; Brewer 1988; McAdoo 1988; National Research Council 1989; Blauner 1989.

3 Unlike white feminist writers who often define themselves in opposition to their mothers, American black women writers since the 1960s have engaged in a celebration of the maternal presence emphasising the generational continuity between mothers and daughters (Washington 1984; Willis 1987; Carby 1987; Hirsch 1989). For a select bibliography of black women's writing in America, see Timberlake *et al.* 1988; Redfern 1989; also Ladner 1972; Lerner 1972; Walker 1974; Rodgers-Rose 1980; Moraga and Anzaldua 1981; Davis 1982; Hull *et al.* 1982; Hooks 1983; Giddings 1984; Steady 1985 (1981); Gray White 1987; Malson *et al.* 1990. For Britain, see Kanter *et al.* 1984; Bhabha *et al.* 1985; Bryan, Dadzie and Scafe 1985; Grewal *et al.* 1988.

4 It has been suggested that Driver sensationalised his findings in a *New Society* article entitled 'How West Indians Do Better at School (Especially the Girls)' (17 Jan. 1980), and that the claims he made could not be substantiated in his study (see Carrington 1981:299).

5 Black girls obtained a mean of 7.6 passes at 'O' level and CSE compared with only a mean of 5.6 for the black boys (Fuller 1982).

6 See Phizacklea (1983:7); Allen (1987:177); Brittan and Maynard (1984:7); Fuller (1982:88), respectively.

7 In the UK issues surrounding invisibility and the various cultural interpretations of 'the family', 'motherhood' and 'marriage' have been the subject of an ongoing black and white socialist feminist debate.

For black British women writers, see Carby 1982b; Anthias and Yuval-Davis 1983; Amos and Parmar 1984; Bhavnani and Coulson 1986; Ramazanoglu *et al.* 1986; Phoenix 1987; Parmar 1989; Bhachu (forthcoming).

For white British women, see Bourne 1983; Barrett and McIntosh 1985; Segal 1987; Ramazanoglu 1989; Ware 1991.

For writings on the development of a black feminist theory in the USA, see Joseph 1981; Joseph and Lewis 1981; Dill 1983; Hooks 1984, 1989,1991; Cole 1986; Collins 1986,1990; Carby 1987; Palmer 1987; Jordan 1989; Malson *et al.* 1990; Spelman 1988; Wall 1990.

For the Caribbean, see Cuales 1988; Reddock 1988; Wiltshire-Brodber 1988; Tang Nain 1991.

8 The Report was first submitted to the DES in 1984. Its release two weeks after the Tottenham uprising was met with a substantial amount of publicity. See: *Guardian*, 17 Oct. 1985, 'Schools Hamper Hopes of Young Blacks'; *Guardian*, 17 Oct. 1985,'The Teachers at the Heart of the Crisis'; *Guardian*, 31 Oct. 1985,'Low Achievement of the Young Pupil is Often the Consequence of the System'.

9 *School Leavers Survey*: see Swann Report (DES 1985); Sillitoe and Meltzer 1985; *Ethnic Background and Examination Results*: Research and Statistics Report 1987 (ILEA/RS/1120/87).

10 The mean performance score for African Caribbean girls was 15.9 compared to 11.2 for the boys, 13.6 for the ESWI boys and 16.9 for the ESWI girls. (ESWI refers to the countries of the British Isles: England, Scotland, Wales and Ireland.)

11 This, however, does not mean that there has not been any 'public' interest in the issue. Recent years have been characterised by a 'sensational' media curiosity with regard to the academic achievement of black girls. For example, a report in the *TES* (3 April 1987) which suggested 'Black Girls Flying High in Reading and Writing', was referring to the findings of a recently published report (Tizard, Blatchford, Burke, Farquhar and Plewis 1988), which among its many conclusions makes only mention of the fact that black girls at the end of infants' school were ahead in their reading and writing skills (p. 180).

3 Do schools make a difference?

1 The names of the two schools, pupils and staff have all been changed.

2 The schools' religious orientation was found to be of immense value. St Hilda's, because of its specific intake drawn from the local Catholic population, provided a unique research opportunity to compare the white, ethnic-minority, second-generation female experience (i.e. Irish) with that of their black counterparts. Likewise the single-sex school situation also enabled me to observe, as a control on the co-educational position, how black females construct their career choices without the influence of male peers.

3 Official reports such as HM Inspectorate Quinquennial Report 1984 (St Hilda's); St Theresa's Quinquennial Review 1977–1982 presented to the Board of Governors.

4 Part of the reason given by Dr Ashraf for the non-response to the racism in his class was the lack of solidarity he felt with the head and his colleagues which stemmed largely from his 'race'.

5 Mortimore *et al.* (ILEA 1986a) suggest that teachers who remain more than seven years in one post reach a point of stagnation. Indeed the teachers who had been there a long time were characterised by their rigidity and inflexibility when it came to change. Several of these teachers were also notable for their racism, suspicion and lack of communication.

6 In the re-organisation of Catholic schools that took place in 1984 (for 1985), Madden re-applied for the post of headmaster but failed to secure his old position.

7 The problems and advantages of single-sex schools are debated in Dale (1974), *Mixed or Single Sex Schools*. There are those that suggest it is of positive benefit, particularly those belonging to the religious lobby, especially Muslims (see Swann Report, DES 1985:504–9). Others, including feminist writers, suggest it has serious drawbacks in some particular contexts, especially with regard to access to systems of power: see Okely (1987).

8 Basil Bernstein (1970) in a *New Society* article considers the issue and concludes that schools cannot do so.

4 Life in the classroom

1 This response of 48% was in marked contrast to their white peers who, in answer to the same question, were far less likely to indicate themselves (e.g., only 25% of white females and 16% of white males indicated that they would like to be like nobody but themselves). Black males, like their female counterparts, were more likely to indicate themselves; i.e. 50%.

2 During the period of my fieldwork (1983–1984), the issue of racism in schools received a great deal of media attention, not least as a result of the publication of the ILEA's Anti-Racist Statements and Policy Guidelines (ILEA 1983), and the controversial activities of the GLC. The various arguments of the anti-racist debate have been documented. For a general appraisal, see Troyna 1987, while Palmer (1986) presents the protagonists' views.

3 It must be noted that this orientation was by no means only found among practising Christians; it was an attitude that extended to non-religious teaching staff and was identified by the philosophy of colour-blindness, not Christian belief.

4 This Newsletter caused outrage among black parents and pupils in the school, who felt it was offensive. One parent, for example, found being likened to French accents and Italian clothes particularly offensive, while others felt it stupid and shallow. Teachers, however, although they too felt it was a rather awkward statement, put it down to the 'hamfisted' eccentricity of Mr Madden and were therefore prepared to overlook it.

5 The MRE Working Party at St Hilda's constantly met with opposition. The Working Party's status was under threat, not least by the head, who felt it was an unnecessary committee. In several instances he went out of his way to obstruct the holding of meetings, giving no time allowances to

the staff involved. He himself only attended one meeting when the Multi-Racial Inspector of the borough came to review the school's progress on the matter.

6 A research study by Rubovits and Maehr (1973) showed that in fact gifted blacks get the least assistance.

7 Further evidence of the girls' need for assistance was illustrated by the fact that their mock results were considerably below average, with many young women absenting themselves rather than fail.

8 Green (DES 1985:52) found that with tolerant teachers who used the indirect teaching method, black girls received more than their fair share of attention and also received less criticism about their work.

9 This shame was not shared by Anita or her boyfriend, who regarded the matter in a totally different light. See Chapter 5.

10 In a similar incident at St Theresa's the pregnancy of a fourth-year black girl was also suppressed.

11 It should also be noted that Ms Wallace was engaged on a part-time MA in Education, and was particularly interested in the issue of gender in schools.

12 As the Destination Questionnaires subsequently showed, Sharon did eventually complete her social work course despite Ms Parker's strong reservations to me four years earlier.

13 Gina was a black fifth-year student at St Hilda's who had a reputation for being particularly difficult, which she was in some ways. However she was prevented from pursuing a number of courses that she showed an interest in because the teachers of those lessons did not want her there. As a consequence she could not do textile design and needlework, two subjects she really wanted to do and was reasonably good at. The rather weak reason put forward by the Textile Design teacher was this: 'She makes no effort in Maths: and Maths and Design are clearly related.'

14 The black teachers appeared to 'share' this common orientation even though they were not all from the same school and thus did not know one another.

15 Ray Rist (1970) comments on the fact that black teachers responded in the class in such a way as to show no difference between black and white pupils.

16 Dr Ashraf had a Ph.D. from India, had completed two years' post-doctoral research at a college of the University of London and had a PGCE.

5 Entering the world of work

1 Lee and Wrench 1983; Austin 1987; OPCS 1987.

2 There were schemes acknowledged to be more prestigious than others. The better the scheme the more likely were pupils to secure employment upon leaving. These schemes were mainly run by large private employers. Those run by local authority employers were less likely to secure a job but were heavily subscribed. Most nursery nursing or care-orientated

choices belonged to this latter category. Austin (1984) notes that Careers officers were under considerable pressure to match trainees to placements as soon as possible.

3 In a bid to stem the growing problem of unemployment and extend the influence of rational manpower planning, the Local Education Authority in partnership with the MSC have developed the TVEI (Technical and Vocational Education Initiative). Courses offered under this Initiative have resulted in the increased involvement of the MSC within schools (see Ainley 1988).

4 The delivery of YTS is structured in many different ways (MSC 1982). In one form it is devolved to organisations known as 'managing agents' (i.e., large firms) who run their own training programmes, which were known as 'mode A' schemes. Where the MSC run their own programmes these are known as 'mode B' schemes. The distinction of schemes into modes A and B has since been abolished, but YTS remains essentially made up of inferior and superior programmes. Since May 1990 YTS has been replaced by YT, administered at local level by TECs (Training and Enterprise Councils). TECs are business-led local companies which contract with the Secretary of State for Employment to take charge of training and enterprise in their area.

5 On the whole, the white boys found careers advice in school most useful compared to any of the other groups designated by race or gender; 88% of white boys indicated that school-based careers advice was useful.

6 For example, nursery nurse, nurse, air hostess, cook, hairdresser.

7 There was a notable difference in occupational aspirations of middle-class white girls (i.e. social classes 1 and 2) compared to working-class girls of other races in the third year. These girls were clearly drawing on their home background as a source of information when making their choices. These early choices already encompassed the expectation that they would be going on to do further studies, often in order to secure a non-traditional female profession. For example, one girl stated that she would 'want to do accounting. My father said to do maths and computing.'

8 With the establishment of the new GCSE exam this problem is even more acute. At the time of my project, GCSE was not yet fully integrated into the curriculum.

9 It should be noted that while doing re-sits some girls were also taking other subjects at other levels too (i.e., first-year 'A' level, GCSE courses, or other vocationally orientated courses such as typing and office skills). However, the main reason for staying on was to re-sit.

10 Craft and Craft (1983) found that black pupils were more likely to apply to polytechnics than to universities.

11 Similarly, Wilson (1987) suggests that the blacks living in the inner city form an 'underclass'. Professional, educated, middle-class blacks move out of these declining areas, leaving behind a residual 'ghetto' culture.

12 This is not to say that black women are ignored. They are mentioned, but

nearly always in terms of their negative reproductive capacity. Wilson (1987), for example, uses as indicators of black social disadvantage the high rates of what he calls 'out of wedlock births' and 'teenage pregnancy'.

13 Even among the young women wishing to pursue further or higher education all chose colleges and polytechnics situated in London; i.e., South Bank Polytechnic, University of London Goldsmiths' College, South London College, Brixton College, Vauxhall College and so on.

14 London Borough of Lambeth (1985:34) notes that a greater proportion of female young unemployed were school leavers: 87% compared to 79% for men. Of young women 47% had been out of work for 6 months or over with 87% being school leavers. Of young men, 49% had been unemployed for over 6 months with 75% being school leavers.

6 Strategic careers

1 The media has also taken a particular interest in the subject (*Guardian*, 12 June 1991; *Voice*, 18 June 1991). Offering a sensational and simplistic interpretation of what are, in effect, complex social phenomena, they mischievously suggest that black women are more 'successful' than their male counter parts.

2 It is interesting to note that 2% of young black women aspired to jobs of a lower social class than they expected. This indicated their wish to do certain 'female'-defined jobs that entailed skills such as cooking or child care which they were aware were thought of as low-status or low-paid. These were clearly desires that they held but did not expect to pursue in the real job market because they felt it was undesirable in the long run to do so.

3 Ullah (1985b), on observing a similar phenomenon, puts forward the explanation that this is because black females, in contrast to black males, do not expect to encounter as much racial discrimination in the labour market.

4 Despite its high status classification (social class 1 and 2), general nursing was not considered as highly as other professional caring jobs. Black nurses are often employed as SENs (State Enrolled Nurses) rather than the more highly qualified SRNs (State Registered Nurses). Because of the West Indian experience in the NHS, and its infamous tradition regarding pay and conditions, it was not thought of as an upwardly mobile choice: specific nursing occupations, such as midwifery, paediatrics and radiography, were more highly regarded.

5 Of the black mothers in the sample population 10% were engaged in the process of re-training (this is in contrast to the white mothers, *none* of whom was similarly engaged). This finding is in line with the national statistics that also suggest that a large number of black women over the age of 24 are in education. See Labour Force Survey (*Employment Gazette* 1987) and Brown 1984.

6 While more opportunities have been made possible by changes in the economy, it must be noted that racism remains a structural problem in this sector in terms of recruitment, promotion, specific access to certain types of job, type of industry and employer prejudice. Thus in many ways what is often regarded as changes that have resulted in greater equality (Wilkie 1985) is an illusion rather than a fact.

7 This tendency is often referred to as 'talent'. 'Talent', however, is a term not chosen to describe these girls' preferences as it implies some form of inherent, genetic capacity or ability for a particular skill.

8 Sport is an area of skill and interest that in relation to black youth has often been attributed to teacher stereotyping and the presence of in- herent, genetic black athleticism. See Cashmore (1981, 1982), Carrington (1983) and Carrington and Wood (1986). Even though females are mentioned by name in these androcentric analyses, sport has yet to be discussed in the context of the 'phenomenon' of high black female aspirations evident for all aspects of educational opportunty.

9 Several studies (Smith 1977; Brown 1984; Ullah 1985a), suggest that compared to young black men and young white men and women, black women are the least aware of racism prior to their entry into the labour market. However, when they do inevitably experience it, they react the most strongly against it.

10 The 'promise', of course, is very different from the reality. There is clear evidence of racial harassment in the armed forces. See, for example, the report: 'Soldier Accuses Army of Racial Discrimination' (*Guardian*, 27 Jan. 1988).

11 Among black pupils 46% (n=33) responded to the follow-up destination questionnaire. Because of non-response the information provided only allowed for a qualitative consideration of the labour-market experiences of the black pupils in the study.

7 Redefining black womanhood

1 For an analysis of black women's literature and writing in America, see Gates (1986); Carby (1987); Willis (1987) Washington (1989); Wall (1990). For Britain see Ngcobo (1988). For the Caribbean see Cudjoe (1990).

2 See, for example the work of McRobbie (1978a, 1978b, 1990); MacDonald (1980); Roberts (1983); Lees (1986); Wallace (1987).

3 The minority who did not see themselves as Irish appeared to have adopted British cultural values. However, their dissociation from Ireland seemed to be because parental ties were not strong rather than any firm desire to be assimilated into the British culture because of shame or stigma attached to being Irish, as Ullah (1985b:313) suggests.

4 While socialist feminists have argued that for white women marriage is a 'psychologically and materially oppressive institution' (Barrett and McIntosh 1982), they state that for the West Indian, marriage is 'no more

than a prestige conferring act' (Phizacklea 1982:100; see also Sharpe 1987:234). The suggestion is that black people 'mimic' the social institutions of the dominant white society. The effect of this widely held racist assumption has been that marriage, the family and male relationships in the West Indian context are dismissed as unimportant in the lives of black women. Caribbean feminists provide evidence to the contrary (Powell 1986).

5 See Phoenix (1988a;1990) for a detailed discussion of early pregnancy among black and white young women.

6 Eggleston *et al.* (1986:95) show African Caribbean boys to be the least likely of all ethnic and white groups to want their wives to stay at home upon having a child. Similarly, research in the USA has shown that black husbands have a 'permissive' attitude to their wives working (Landry and Jendrek 1978).

7 It is also a common feature of black American life. The literature on the black condition in the USA describes what *in essence* are male–female relationships of relative autonomy and independence between the sexes (Billingsley 1968; Gutman 1976; Ladner 1985; Stack 1974, 1985; Jones 1986; Wilson 1987). However, such relationships are often misunderstood and deemed 'pathological' and thus negative.

8 A clear example of what is meant by misrepresentation is shown in a recent *New Society* article (Williams 1986). In a national survey of young people's attitudes, it was found, in sharp contrast to white youth, that the majority of young West Indian men were willing to share household tasks equally with their partners. Rather than seeing the value of such a finding, the authors are quick to dismiss it as a 'blip' in the results. They suggest the cause of the 'blip' is 'the result of [the boys] observing too many hard-pressed mums'.

9 Research in the USA suggests that among black working wives the husbands' approval did not affect their satisfaction with work (Harrison and Minor 1978).

10 Sutton and Makiesky-Barrow (1977:317) suggest that while much of the literature on sex roles views the domestic sphere as an area of confinement that is associated with women and their dependent status, for the slave population, the domestic area was the one area of life that for both sexes was associated with human freedom and autonomy. See also Mathurin Mair (1986); Wiltshire-Brodber (1988); Bush (1990).

8 Family matters

1 In my study 59% of the working-class West Indian households lived in owner-occupied homes, compared to only 26% of the white working-class families. The white families were far more likely to live in council homes: 64% compared to only 34% of black families.

2 For example, these jobs are classified as lower-status occupations (i.e., office/administrative work is grouped as SC3NM, or trained nursery nurses as SC3M).

3 There have been attempts to incorporate women into a classification schema. For example, Helen Roberts (1987) presents the 'City Classification Scheme' which takes on board the feminist critique of stratification analysis, by her recognition of the domestic responsibility among women hitherto invisible in the economy (see also Acker 1973; Delphy 1981; Delphy and Leonard 1986).

4 In this study the social status of the women who were 'heads of household' was higher than that of the males. Of West Indian women classified as 'head of household' 68% were in social class 1 and 2, whereas only 15% of black males were. The majority of black males who were 'heads of household' were in social class 3, manual occupations (i.e., 46%).

5 The parents' commitment to the labour market was judged by work characteristics such as if they engaged in full-time work or part-time work. Other aspects, such as distance travelled to work, helped to assess their level of involvement in the labour market. With a more adequate questionnaire administered to the parents (and not to the children, as this was) such aspects of length of employment and time off work for child rearing could be included.

6 For example, parents often had 'conservative' social values particularly when it came to such matters as intermarriage and family respect. Many second-generation girls with their experiences of being black British wished to challenge many of what were often regarded as redundant values, as the following statement suggests:

> If I was to bring a dreadlock home, my mother go mad! She'd say, 'He not decent; what will the family think!'...My mum is more against a Rasta than a white boy, but it's not about the colour or the hair but what a person is like.

> (Merle)

7 See Justus (1985) on the central role of the Church in West Indian society. Tomlinson (1983b:73) also notes the influence of the Church and God on black female aspirations in higher education.

8 In answer to the question, 'Who do you most admire?', 49% of the girls in the sample said that the person they admired most was themselves. This was in contrast to their white peers, only 25% of whom gave this answer.

9 With regard to standards of teaching and classroom reactions, in particular the girls in the lower streams felt classes were often a form of containment. One girl explained:

> I am sure if you put the black kids in the high groups they would work but as they put blacks in a low group they will be bound to do no work. I have been streamed low when I know I could do better.

> (Gina)

10 Some teachers were respected and admired by the girls. The reponse to these lessons was markedly different from those the girls did not regard as 'good teachers'.

Bibliography

Abbott, P. and Sapsford, R. (1987) *Women and Social Class*. London, Tavistock.

Acker, J. (1973) 'Women and Social Stratification: a Case of Intellectual Sexism', *American Journal of Sociology*, 78.

Adelman, C. (1985) 'Who Are You? Some Problems of Ethnographer Culture Shock.' In R.G. Burgess (ed.) *Field Methods in the Study of Education*. Brighton: Falmer Press.

Ainley, P. (1988) *From School to YTS: Education and Training in England and Wales 1944–1987*. Milton Keynes: Open University Press.

Alba, R.D. (ed.) (1985) *Ethnicity and Race in the USA: Toward the Twenty-First Century*. London: Routledge and Kegan Paul.

Allen, S. (1982) 'Confusing Categories and Neglecting Contradictions'. In E. Cashmore and B. Troyna (eds) *Black Youth in Crisis*. London: George Allen & Unwin.

—— (1987) 'Gender, Race, and Class in the 1980s'. In C. Husband (ed.) *Race in Britain, Continuity and Change: The Second Edition*. London: Hutchinson.

Allen, S. and Smith, C.R. (1975) 'Minority Group Experience in the Transition from Education to Work'. In P. Branner (ed.) *Entering the World of Work: Some Sociological Perspectives*. Department of Employment, London: HMSO.

Amos, V. and Parmar, P. (1981) 'Resistances and Responses: Experiences of Black Girls in Britain'. In A. McRobbie and T. McCabe (eds) *Feminism for Girls: An Adventure Story*. London: Routledge and Kegan Paul.

—— (1984) 'Challenging Imperial Feminism.' *Feminist Review*. Special issue: Many Voices One Chant, Black Feminist Perspectives, 17 (Autumn).

Anthias, F. and Yuval-Davis, N. (1983) 'Contextualizing Feminism: Gender, Ethnic and Class Divisions'. *Feminist Review*, 15 (Winter).

Austin, R.J. (1984) 'Black Girls in the Youth Training Scheme'. Dissertation for M.Sc. in Race and Ethnic Relations. Research Unit on Ethnic Relations: University of Aston, Birmingham.

—— (1987) 'YTS, Black Girls and the Careers Service'. In M. Cross and D.I.

Smith (eds) *Black Youth Futures: Ethnic Minorities and the Youth Training Scheme*. Leicester: National Youth Bureau.

Bagley, C., Bart, M. and Wong, J. (1979) 'Antecedents of Scholastic Success in West Indian Ten Year Olds in London'. In G.K. Verma and C. Bagley (eds) *Race, Education and Identity*. London: Macmillan.

Bagley, C., Mallick, K. and Verma, G.K. (1979) 'Pupil Self-esteem – a Study of Black and White Teenagers in British Schools'. In G.K. Verma and C. Bagley (eds) *Race, Education and Identity*. London: Macmillan.

Bagley, C. and Verma, G. (1980) 'Brimer Wide-Span Reading Scores in Pupils Aged 14–16 Years in English Secondary Schools'. Unpublished paper, University of Surrey.

Banks, M., Ullah, P. and Warr, P. (1984) 'Unemployment and Less Qualified Urban Young People'. *Employment Gazette*, 92 (Aug.): 343–6.

Barrett, M. and McIntosh, M. (1982) *The Anti-social Family*. London: Verso.

—— (1985) 'Ethnocentrism and Socialist-Feminist Theory'. *Feminist Review*, 20 (Summer).

Barron, R.D. and Norris, G.M. (1976) 'Sexual Divisions and the Dual Labour Market'. In D. Barker and S. Allen (eds) *Sexual Divisions in Society: Process and Change*. London: Tavistock.

Barrow, C. (1986) 'Finding Support: Strategies for Survival'. *Social and Economic Studies*, Special No.: J. Massiah (ed.) *Women in the Caribbean* (Part 1): Institute of Social and Economic Research, Cave Hill: University of the West Indies, 35 (2).

—— (1988) 'Anthropology, the Family and Women in the Caribbean'. In P. Mohammed and C. Shepherd *Gender in Caribbean Development*. Women and Development Studies Project, St Augustine, Trinidad: University of the West Indies.

Beale, J. (1986) *Women in Ireland*. London: Macmillan.

Beechey, V. (1978) 'Women and Production: A Critical Analysis of Some Sociological Theories of Women's Work'. In A. Khun and A.M. Wolpe (eds) *Feminism and Materialism*. London: Routledge and Kegan Paul.

—— (1987) *Unequal Work*. London: Verso.

Beechey, V. and Perkins, T. (1987) *A Matter of Hours: Women, Part-time Work and the Labour Market*. London: Polity.

Benyon, J. and Solomos, J. (eds) (1987) *The Roots of Urban Unrest*. Oxford: Pergamon Press.

Bernstein, B. (1970) 'Education Cannot Compensate for Society'. *New Society*, 26 Feb.

Bettelheim, B. and Janowitz, M. (1977) 'The Consequences of Social Mobility'. In J. Stone (ed.) *Race, Ethnicity, and Social Change*. North Scituate, Mass.: Duxbury Press.

Bhabha, J., Klug, F. and Shutter, S. (eds) (1985) *Worlds Apart: Women under Immigration and Nationality Law*. London: Pluto Press.

Bhachu, P. (1986) 'Work, Dowry, and Marriage among East African Sikh Women in the United Kingdom'. In R.J. Simon and C.B. Brettell (eds)

International Migration: The Female Experience. Totowa, NJ: Rowman & Allenheld.

—— (1991) 'Culture, Ethnicity and Class among Punjabi Sikh Women in 1990s Britain'. *New Community*, 17 (3) (April).

—— (forthcoming) 'Identities Constructed and Reconstructed: Asian Women in Britain'. In J. Buigs and S. Ardner (eds) *Women Crossing Boundaries: Dilemmas of Changing Identities.* Oxford: Berg Press.

Bhavnani, K. (1989) 'Complexity, Activism, and Optimism', *Feminist Review*, 31.

—— (1991) *Talking Politics: A Psychological Framing for Views from Youth in Britain.* Cambridge: Cambridge University Press.

Bhavnani, K. and Coulson, M. (1986) 'Transforming Socialist Feminism: The Challenge of Racism'. *Feminist Review*, 23: 81–92.

Billingsley, A. (1968) *Black Families in White America.* Englewood Cliffs, NJ: Prentice-Hall.

Blackburn, R. and Mann, M. (1981) 'Ethnic Stratification in an Industrial City'. In P. Braham, E. Rhodes and M. Pearn (eds) *Discrimination and Disadvantage in Employment.* London: Harper & Row in association with the Open University.

Blauner, R. (1989) *Black Lives, White Lives: Three Decades of Race Relations in America.* California: University of California Press.

Bonacich, E. (1979) 'The Past, Present and Future of Split Labour Market Theory'. *Research in Race and Ethnic Relations*, 1.

Boudon, R. (1973) *Education, Opportunity and Social Inequality.* New York: John Wiley & Sons.

—— (1977) 'Education and Social Mobility'. In J. Karabel and A.H. Halsey (eds) *Power and Ideology in Education.* New York: Oxford University Press.

Bourdieu, P. (1973) 'Cultural Reproduction and Social Reproduction'. In R. Brown (ed.) *Knowledge, Education, and Cultural Change.* London: Tavistock.

—— (1977) 'Cultural Reproduction and Social Reproduction'. In J. Karabel and A.H. Halsey (eds) *Power and Ideology in Education.* New York: Oxford University Press.

Bourne, J. (1983) 'Towards an Anti-Racist Feminism'. *Race and Class*, 25 (1).

Bowles, S. (1977) 'Unequal Education and the Reproduction of the Social Division of Labour'. In J. Karabel and A.H. Halsey (eds) *Power and Ideology in Education.* New York: Oxford University Press.

Brah, A. (1988) 'Extended Review: Gender and the Politics of Schooling'. *British Journal of Sociology*, 9 (1).

Brake, M. (1990; 1st edition, 1985) *Comparative Youth Culture: The Sociology of Youth Subcultures in America, Britain and Canada.* London: Routledge.

Brewer, R. (1988) 'Black Women in Poverty: Some Comments on Female-Headed Families'. *Signs: Journal of Women in Culture and Society*, 13 (2).

Brewer, R.I. and Haslum, M.N. (1986) 'Ethnicity: The Experience of Socio-economic Disadvantage and Educational Attainment'. *British Journal of Sociology of Education*, 7 (1).

Brittan, A. and Maynard, M. (1984) *Sexism, Racism and Oppression*. Oxford: Basil Blackwell.

Britten, N. and Heath, A. (1983) 'Women, Men and Social Class'. In E. Gamarnikow (ed.) *Gender, Class and Work*. London: Heinemann.

Brooks, D. (1983) 'Young Blacks and Asians in the Labour Market: A Critical Overview'. In B. Troyna and D.I. Smith (eds) *Racism, School and the Labour Market*. Leicester: National Youth Bureau.

Brown, C. (1984) *Black and White in Britain: The Third PSI Survey*. London: Heinemann.

Brown, P. (1987) *Schooling Ordinary Kids: Inequality, Unemployment, and the New Vocationalism*. London: Tavistock.

Browne, M. (1981) *Careers Opportunities and Education*. Manchester: Equal Opportunities Commission.

Bryan, B., Dadzie, S. and Scafe, S. (1985) *The Heart of the Race: Black Women's Lives in Britain*. London: Virago.

Bullivant, B.M. (1982) 'Power and Control in the Multi-ethnic School: Towards a Conceptual Model'. *Ethnic and Racial Studies*, 5 (2): 54–70.

Burney, E. (1988) *Steps to Racial Equality: Positive Action in a Negative Climate*. London: The Runnymede Trust.

Bush, B. (1990) *Slave Women in Caribbean Society 1650–1838*. London: James Currey.

Carby, H.V. (1982a) 'Schooling in Babylon'. In Centre for Contemporary Cultural Studies *The Empire Strikes Back: Race and Racism in Seventies Britain*. London: Hutchinson.

—— (1982b) 'White Woman Listen! Black Feminism and the Boundaries of Sisterhood'. In Centre for Contemporary Cultural Studies *The Empire Strikes Back: Race and Racism in Seventies Britain*. London: Hutchinson.

—— (1987) (ed.) *Reconstructing Womanhood: The Emergence of the Afro-American Woman Novelist*. New York: Oxford University Press.

Carrington, B. (1981) 'Schooling an Underclass: The Implications of Ethnic Differences in Attainment'. *Durham and Newcastle Research Reviews*, 9 (47) (Autumn).

—— (1983) 'Sport as a Side Track. An Analysis of Extra-curricular Sport'. In L. Barton and S. Walker (eds) *Race, Class and Education*. Beckenham, Kent: Croom Helm.

Carrington, B. and Wood, E. (1986) 'Black Youth and Sport in the United Kingdom'. In C. Brock (ed.) *The Caribbean in Europe*. London: Frank Cass.

Cashmore, E. (1981) 'The Black British Sporting Life'. *New Society*, 57 (977).

—— (1982) *Black Sportsmen*. London: Routledge and Kegan Paul.

Cashmore, E. and Troyna, B. (1982) *Black Youth in Crisis*. London: George Allen & Unwin.

Central Statistical Office (1991) *Social Trends 21*. London: HMSO.

Centre for Contemporary Cultural Studies (1981) *Unpopular Education: Schooling and Social Democracy in England since 1944*. London: Hutchinson.

Chevannes, M. (1979) 'The Black Arrow Supplementary School Project'. *The Social Science Teacher*, 8 (4).

Chevannes, M. and Reeves, F. (1987) 'The Black Voluntary School Movement: Definition, Context and Prospects.' In B. Troyna (ed.) *Racial Inequality in Education*. London: Tavistock.

Chigwada, R. (1987) 'Not Victims – Not Superwomen'. *Spare Rib*, 183.

Chivers, T.S. (1987) *Race and Culture in Education*. Windsor: NFER–Nelson.

Chodorow, N. (1979) 'Mothering, Male Dominance, and Capitalism'. In Z.R. Eisenstein (ed.) *Capitalist Patriarchy and the Case for Socialist Feminism*. New York: Monthly Review Press.

Cicourel, A.V. and Kitsuse, J.I. (1977) 'The School as a Mechanism of Social Differentiation'. In J. Karabel and A.H. Halsey (eds) *Power and Ideology in Education*. New York: Oxford University Press.

Clark, R.M. (1983) *Family Life and School Achievement: Why Poor Black Children Succeed or Fail*. Chicago: University of Chicago Press.

Clarke, E. (1975: 1st edition, 1957) *My Mother Who Fathered Me*. London: George Allen & Unwin.

Clarke, L. (1980) *The Transition from School to Work: A Critical Review of Research in the United Kingdom*. London: Department of Employment, Careers Service Branch, HMSO.

Coard, B. (1971) *How the West Indian Child Is Made ESN in the British School System*. London: New Beacon Books.

Cockburn, C. (1987) *Two Track Training*. London: Tavistock.

Cole, J. (1986) *All American Woman: Lines That Divide, Ties That Bind*. New York: The Free Press.

Coleman, J.S. (1960) 'The Adolescent Sub-Culture and Academic Achievement'. *American Journal of Sociology*, 65 (Jan.): 337–47.

Coleman, J.S., Campbell, E., Hobson, C., McPortland, J., Mood, A., Weinfeld, F. and York, R. (1969) *Equality of Educational Opportunity*. Cambridge, Mass.: Harvard University Press.

Coles, B. and Maynard, M. (1990) 'Moving Towards a Fair Start: Equal Gender Opportunities and the Careers Service'. *Gender and Education*, 2 (3).

Collins, Hill P. (1986) 'Learning from the Outsider Within: The Sociological Significance of Black Feminist Thought'. *Social Problems*, 33 (6).

—— (1990) *Black Feminist Thought*. London: Unwin Hyman.

The Combahee River Collective (1982) 'A Black Feminist Statement'. In G.T. Hull, P.B. Scott and B. Smith (eds) *All the Women Are White, All the Blacks Are Men, but Some of Us Are Brave*. New York: The Feminist Press.

Coopersmith, S. (1975) 'Self-Concept Race and Education'. In G.K. Verma and C. Bagley (eds) *Race and Education Across Cultures*. London: Heinemann.

Coultas, V. (1989) 'Black Girls and Self-esteem'. *Gender and Education*,

Special Issue: Race, Gender and Education, O. Foster-Carter and C. Wright (eds), 1 (3).

Cowie, L. and Lees, S. (1981) 'Slags or Drags'. *Feminist Review*, 9: 17–31.

Craft, M. and Craft, A. (1983) 'The Participation of Ethnic Minority Pupils in Further and Higher Education'. *Educational Research*, 25 (1) (Feb).

Crompton, R. and Mann, M. (eds) (1986) *Gender and Stratification*. Cambridge: Polity Press.

Cross, M. (1986) 'Migration and Exclusion: Caribbean Echoes and British Realities'. In C. Brock (ed.) *The Caribbean in Europe: Aspects of the West Indian Experience in Britain, France and the Netherlands*. London: Frank Cass.

—— (1987a) 'Who Goes Where? Placement of Black Youth on YTS'. In M. Cross and D.I. Smith (eds) *Black Youth Futures: Ethnic Minorities and the Youth Training Scheme*. Leicester: National Youth Bureau.

—— (1987b) 'Generation Jobless: The Need for a New Agenda in Ethnic Relations Policy'. *New Community*, 15 (1/2) (Autumn).

—— (1987c) 'Equality of Opportunity and Inequality of Outcome: The MSC, Ethnic Minorities and Training Policy'. In R. Jenkins and J. Solomos (eds) *Racism and Equal Opportunity Policies in the 1980s*. Cambridge: Cambridge University Press.

—— (1988) 'Mobility Denied: Afro-Caribbean Labour and the British Economy'. In M. Cross and H. Entzinger (eds) *Lost Illusions: Caribbean Minorities in Britain and the Netherlands*. London: Routledge.

Cross, M. and Johnson, M. (forthcoming) 'Race and the Urban System'. Paper presented to the Postgraduate Seminar, Goldsmiths' College, University of London, 1988.

Cuales, S. (1988) 'Some Theoretical Considerations on Social Class, Class Consciousness and Gender Consciousness'. In P. Mohammed and C. Shepherd *Gender in Caribbean Development*. Women and Development Studies Project, St Augustine, Trinidad: University of the West Indies.

Cudjoe, S.R. (ed.) (1990) *Caribbean Women Writers: Essays from the First International Conference*, Wellesley, Mass.: Calaloux Publications.

Currie, D. and Kazi, H. (1987) 'Academic Feminism and the Process of De-radicalization: Re-examining the issues'. *Feminist Review*, 25 (Spring).

Dale, R. (1974) *Mixed or Single Sex School: Attainment, Attitudes and Overview*, Vol. 3, London: Routledge and Kegan Paul.

Dann, G. (1987) *The Barbadian Male: Sexual Attitudes and Practice*. London: Macmillan.

David, M.E. (1989) 'Education'. In M. McCarthy (ed.) *The New Politics of Welfare: An Agenda for the 1990s*. London: Macmillan.

Davis, A. (1982) *Women, Race and Class*. London: The Women's Press.

Davis, A. and Davis, F. (1986) 'The Black Family and the Crisis of Capitalism'. *The Black Scholar*, 17 (5).

Davison, R.B. (1966) *Black British: Immigrants to England*. London: Oxford University Press and the Institute of Race Relations.

Dawson, A. (1988) 'Inner City Adolescents: Unequal Attainments'. In G.

Verma and P. Pumfrey (eds) *Educational Attainments*. East Sussex: Falmer Press.

Deakin, N. (1970) *Colour, Citizenship and British Society*. London: Panther.

Delamont, S. (1980) *Sex Roles and the School*. London: Methuen.

Delphy, C. (1981) 'Women in Stratification Studies'. In H. Roberts (ed.) *Doing Feminist Research*. London: Routledge and Kegan Paul.

Delphy, C. and Leonard, D. (1986) 'Class Analysis, Gender Analysis and the Family'. In R. Crompton and M. Mann (eds) *Gender and Stratification*. London: Polity Press.

Department of Education and Science (1973) *Careers Education in Secondary Schools*. Education Survey 18, London: HMSO.

—— (1981) *West Indian Children in Our Schools: A Report of the Committee of Inquiry into the Education of Children from Ethic Minority Groups*. The Rampton Report, HMSO, Cmnd 8273.

—— (1985) *Education for All: The Report of the Committee of Inquiry into the Education of Children from Ethnic Minority Groups*. The Swann Report, HMSO, Cmnd 9453.

Dex, S. (1982) 'West Indians, Further Education and Labour Markets'. *New Community*, 10 (2) (Winter): 191–205.

—— (1983) 'The Second Generation: West Indian Female School Leavers'. In A. Phizacklea (ed.) *One Way Ticket*. London: Routledge and Kegan Paul.

—— (1985) *The Sexual Division of Labour*. Brighton, Sussex: Wheatsheaf Books.

Dhondy, F., Beese, B. and Hassan, L. (1974) *The Black Explosion in British Schools*. London: Race Today Publications.

Dill, Thornton B. (1980) 'The Means to Put My Children Through: Child Rearing Strategies Among Black Female Domestic Servants'. In L. Rogers-Rose (ed.) *The Black Woman*. Beverly Hills, Cal.: Sage.

—— (1983) 'Race, Class, and Gender: Prospects for an All-Inclusive Sisterhood'. *Feminist Studies*, 9 (1).

—— (1990) 'The Dialectics of Black Womanhood'. In M. Malson, E. Mudimbe-Boyi, J. O'Barr and M. Wyer *Black Women in America: Social Science Perspectives*. Chicago: University of Chicago Press.

Dodgson, E. (1984) *Motherland: West Indian Women to Britain in the 1950s*. Oxford: Heinemann Educational Books.

Dove, L. (1975) 'The Hopes of Immigrant School Children'. *New Society*, 32: 63–5.

Drew, D. and Gray, J. (1991) 'The Black and White Gap in Examination Results: A Statistical Critique of a Decade of Research'. *New Community*, 17 (2).

Driver, G. (1977) 'Cultural Competence, Social Power and School Achievement'. *New Community*, 5 (4).

—— (1979) 'Classroom Stress and School Achievement: West Indian Adolescents and Their Teachers'. In V.S. Khan (ed.) *Minority Families in Britain*. London: Macmillan.

—— (1980a) 'How West Indians Do Better at School (Especially the Girls)'. *New Society*, 17 Jan.

—— (1980b) *Beyond Underachievement: Case Studies of English, West Indian and Asian School Leavers at Sixteen Plus*. London: Commission for Racial Equality.

—— (1982) 'Ethnicity and Cultural Competence: Aspects of Interaction in Multi-Racial Classrooms'. In G.K. Verma and C. Bagley (eds) *Self-Concept, Achievement and Multi-Cultural Education*. London: Macmillan.

Durant-Gonzalez, V. (1982) 'The Realm of Female Familial Responsibility'. In J. Massiah (ed.) *Women in the Caribbean Research Papers*, Vol. 2: *Women and the Family*. Cave Hill, Barbados: Institute of Social and Economic Research, University of the West Indies.

Eggleston, J., Dunn, D., Anjali, M. and Wright, C. (1986) *Education for Some. The Educational and Vocational Experiences of 15–18 Year Old Members of Minority Ethnic Groups*, Stoke-on-Trent: Trentham.

Ellis, P. (1986) 'Education and a Woman's Place in Caribbean Society'. In P. Ellis (ed.) *Women of the Caribbean*. London: Zed Books.

Equal Opportunities Commission (1990) *The Key to Real Choice*. Manchester: EOC.

Employment Gazette (1985) 'Ethnic Origin and Economic Status'. London: Department of Employment (Dec.), HMSO.

—— (1987) 'Ethnic Origin and Economic Status'. London: Department of Employment (Jan.), HMSO.

—— (1990) 'Ethnic Origins and the Labour Market'. London: Department of Employment (March), HMSO.

—— (1991) 'Ethnic Origins and the Labour Market'. London: Department of Employment (Feb.), HMSO.

Farley, R. (1984) *Blacks and Whites. Narrowing the Gap?* Cambridge, Mass.: Harvard University Press.

—— (1985) 'Three Steps Forward and Two Steps Back? Recent Changes in the Social and Economic Status of Blacks'. In R. Alba (ed.) *Ethnicity and Race in the USA: Toward the Twenty-first Century*. Boston, Mass.: Routledge and Kegan Paul.

Farley, R. and Bianchi, S.M. (1985) 'Social Class Polarisation: Is It Occurring Among the Blacks?' In M. Leggon, *Research in Race and Ethnic Relations*, 4: 1–31.

Farnham, C. (1987) 'Sapphire? The Issue of Dominance in the Slave Family'. In C. Groneman and M. Norton *To Toil the Live Long Day: America's Women at Work*. Ithaca, NY: Cornell University Press.

Figueroa, P. (1976) 'The Employment Prospects of West Indian School Leavers in London, England'. *Social and Economic Studies*, 25: 216–23.

Fitzherbert, K. (1967) *West Indian Children in London*. London: Bell & Sons.

Flude, M. and Hammer, M. (eds) (1989) *The 1988 Education Reform Act*. Barcombe: Falmer Press.

Fogelman, K. (1983) *Growing Up in Great Britain*. London: Macmillan.

Foner, N. (1979) *Jamaica Farewell: Jamaican Migrants in London*. London: Routledge and Kegan Paul.

Foster, E. (1988) 'Black Girls and Pastoral Care'. In C. Duncan *Pastoral Care: An Anti-Racist/Multi-Cultural Perspective*. Oxford: Basil Blackwell.

Fowler, B., Littlewood, B. and Madigan, R. (1977) 'Immigrant School Leavers and the Search for Work'. *Sociology*, 11 (2).

Frazier, E.F. (1966) *The Negro Family in the United States*. Chicago: University of Chicago Press.

Fryer, P. (1984) *Staying Power: The History of Black People in Britain*. London: Pluto.

Fuller, M. (1978) 'Dimensions of Gender in a School'. Unpublished Ph.D. thesis, University of Bristol.

—— (1980) 'Black Girls in a London Comprehensive School'. In R. Deem (ed.) *Schooling for Women's Work*. London: Routledge and Kegan Paul.

—— (1982) 'Young, Female and Black'. In E. Cashmore and B. Troyna (eds) *Black Youth in Crisis*. London: George Allen & Unwin.

—— (1983) 'Qualified Criticism, Critical Qualifications'. In L. Barton and S. Walker (eds) *Race, Class and Education*. Beckenham, Kent: Croom Helm.

Gambetta, D. (1988) *Were They Pushed or Did They Jump? Individual Decision Mechanisms in Education*. Cambridge: Cambridge University Press.

Gaskell, G. and Smith, P. (1981) 'Are Young Blacks Really Alienated?' *New Society*, 14 May.

Gates, H.L. (ed.) (1986) *'Race', Writing, and Difference*. Chicago: University of Chicago Press.

Geschwender, J. and Carroll-Seguin, R. (1990) 'Exploding the Myth of African-American Progress in American Society'. In M. Malson, E. Mudimbe-Boyi, J. O'Barr and M. Wyer (eds) *Black Women in America: Social Science Perspectives*. Chicago: University of Chicago Press.

Gibson, A., with J. Barrow (1986) *The Unequal Struggle: The Findings of a West Indian Research Investigation into the Underachievement of West Indian Children in British Schools*. London: The Centre for Caribbean Studies.

Giddings, P. (1984) *Where and When I Enter: The Impact of Race and Sex in America*. New York: Bantam Books.

Giles, R. (1977) *The West Indian Experience in British Schools*. London: Heinemann.

Gill, M. (1984) 'Women, Work and Development in Barbados, 1946–1970'. In J. Massiah (ed.) *Women in the Caribbean Research Papers*, vol. 6: *Women, Work and Development*. Cave Hill, Barbados: Institute of Social and Economic Research, University of the West Indies.

Gilroy, P. (1981) 'You Can't Fool the Youths: Race and Class Formation in the 1980s'. *Race and Class*, 23 (2–3).

—— (1982) 'Steppin' Out of Babylon – Race, Class and Autonomy'. In Centre for Contemporary Cultural Studies *The Empire Strikes Back: Race and Racism in Seventies Britain*. London: Hutchinson.

—— (1987) *There Ain't No Black in the Union Jack*. London: Hutchinson.

—— (1990) 'The End of Anti-racism'. *New Community*, 17 (1) (Oct.).

Glasgow, D. (1981) *The Black Underclass: Poverty, Unemployment and the Entrapment of Ghetto Youth*. New York: Vintage.

Glazer, N. and Moynihan, D.P. (1963) *Beyond the Melting Pot: The Negroes, Puerto Ricans, Jews, Italians and Irish of New York City*. Cambridge, Mass.: MIT Press.

—— (1977) 'A Resurgence of Ethnicity?' In J. Stone (ed.) *Race, Ethnicity, and Social Change*. North Scituate, Mass.: Duxbury Press.

Goldthorpe, J.H. (1983) 'Women and Class Analysis: In Defence of the Conventional View'. *Sociology*, 17.

Goldthorpe, J., Llewellyn, C. and Payne, C. (1988) *Social Mobility and Class Structure in Modern Britain*. 2nd edition. London: Clarendon Press.

Gonzalez, N.S. (1985) 'Household and the Family in the Caribbean: Some Definitions and Concepts'. F.C. Steady (ed.) *The Black Woman Cross-Culturally*. Cambridge, Mass.: Schenkman Books.

Graham, P. and Meadows, C.E. (1967) 'Psychiatric Disorders in the Children of West Indian Immigrants'. *Journal of Child Psychology and Psychiatry*, 8.

Granovetter, M.F. (1973) 'The Strengths of Weak Ties', *American Journal of Sociology*, 78 (6).

Gray White, D. (1987) *Ar'n't I a Woman*. New York: Norton.

Greater London Council (1985) *London: Facts and Figures*. London: Intelligence Unit, Greater London Council (Sept.).

Green, P. (1985) 'Multi-ethnic Teaching and the Pupils' Self-concepts'. In DES 1985, *Education for All* (The Swann Report). HMSO, Cmnd 9453.

Grewal, S., Kay, J., Landor, L., Lewis, G. and Parmar, P. (1988) *Charting a Journey: Writings of Black and Third World Women*. London: Sheba Press.

Griffin, C. (1985) *Typical Girls? Young Women from School to the Job Market*. London: Routledge and Kegan Paul.

—— (1987) 'Broken Transitions: From School to the Scrap Heap'. In P. Allatt, T. Keil, A. Bryman and B. Bytheway (eds) *Women and the Life-cycle Approach*. London: Macmillan.

Gutman, H. (1976) *The Black Family in Slavery and Freedom 1750–1925*. New York: Vintage Books.

Hall, S. (1978) 'Racism and Reaction'. In *Five Views of Multi-racial Britain*. London: Commission for Racial Equality.

Hall, S. and Jefferson, T. (eds) (1976) *Resistance through Rituals: Youth Sub-cultures in Post-war Britain*. London: Hutchinson.

Halsey, A.H. (1972) *Educational Priority Problems and Policies*, No. 1, London: HMSO.

—— (1977) 'Towards Meritocracy? The Case of Britain'. In J. Karabel and A.H. Halsey (eds) *Power and Ideology in Education*. New York: Oxford University Press.

Halsey, A.H., Heath, A.F. and Ridge, J.M. (1980) *Origins and Destinations: Family, Class and Education in Modern Britain*. Oxford: Clarendon Press.

Hannerz, U. (1969) *Soulside: Enquiries into Ghetto Culture and Community*. New York: Columbia University Press.

Hare, N. and Hare, J. (1984) *The Endangered Black Family*. San Francisco: Black Think Tank.

Hargreaves, D. (1976; 1st edition, 1967) *Social Relations in a Secondary School*. London: Routledge and Kegan Paul.

—— (1984) 'Establishing a Common Curriculum'. Paper presented to the School of Education, University of London, Goldsmiths' College, 22 May 1984.

Harrison, A. and Minor, J. (1978) 'Interrole Conflict, Coping Strategies, and Satisfaction Among Black Working Wives'. *Journal of Marriage and the Family* (Nov.).

Hartmann, H. (1979) 'Capitalism, Patriarchy and Job Segregation by Sex'. In Z.R. Eisenstein (ed.) *Capitalist Patriarchy and the Case for Socialist Feminism*. New York: Monthly Review Press.

Heath, A. and Ridge, J. (1983) 'Schools, Examinations and Occupational Attainment'. In J. Purvis and M. Hales (eds) *Achievement and Inequality in Education*. London: Routledge and Kegan Paul.

Heath, A.F. (1987) 'Class in the Classroom'. *New Society* (17 July).

Hebdige, D. (1979) *Subcultures: The Meaning of Style*. London: Methuen.

Hewitt, R. (1986) *White Talk Black Talk: Inter-racial Friendship and Communication Amongst Adolescents*. Cambridge: Cambridge University Press.

Hirsch, M. (1989) *The Mother/Daughter Plot: Narrative, Psychoanalysis, Feminism*. Bloomington, Ind.: Indiana University Press.

Hoch, P. (1979) *White Hero, Black Beast*. London: Pluto.

Hoggart, R. (1957) *The Uses of Literacy*. London: Chatto & Windus.

Holland, J. (1983; 1st edition, 1980) *Work and Women*. Bedford Way Papers, No. 6. Institute of Education, University of London.

Holland, J. and Skouras, G. (1979) *Study of Adolescents' Views of Aspects of the Social Division of Labour*. Social Science Research Council Report, No. 6.

Hooks, B. (1983; 1st edition, 1982) *Ain't I a Woman: Black Women and Feminism*. London: Pluto Press.

—— (1984) *Feminist Theory: From Margin to Centre*. Boston, Mass.: South End Press.

—— (1989) *Talking Back: Thinking Feminist – Thinking Black*. London: Sheba.

—— (1991) 'Sisterhood: Political Solidarity between Women'. In S. Gunew (ed.) *A Reader in Feminist Knowledge*. London: Routledge.

Houghton, V.P. (1966) 'A Report on the Scores of West Indian Immigrant Children and English Children on an Individually Administered Test'. Race, 8 (1).

Hudson, B. (1984) 'Femininity and Adolescence'. In A. McRobbie and M. Nava (eds) *Gender and Generation*. London: Macmillan.

Hull, G.T., Scott, P.B. and Smith B. (eds) (1982) *All the Women Are White, All the Blacks Are Men, But Some of Us Are Brave*. New York: The Feminist Press.

Husband, C. (1987) 'British Racisms: The Construction of Racial Ideologies'. In C. Husband (ed.) *Race in Britain, Continuity and Change: The Second Edition*. London: Hutchinson.

Husen, T. (1977) 'Academic Performance in Selective and Comprehensive Schools'. In J. Karabel and A.H. Halsey (eds) *Power and Ideology in Education*. New York: Oxford University Press.

Inner London Education Authority (1983) *Race, Sex and Class*, (Nos 1–6). London: Inner London Education Authority.

—— (1986a) *The Junior School Project*. London: Research and Statistics Branch, ILEA.

—— (1986b) *Investigating Gender in Schools: A Series of In-Service Workshops for ILEA Teachers* (385/1135m/MH (4)).

—— (1987) *Ethnic Background and Examination Results*. London: Research and Statistics (ILEA/RS/1120/87).

Jackson, B. and Marsden, D. (1963) *Education and the Working Class*. London: Routledge and Kegan Paul.

Jackson, J.A. (1963) *The Irish in Britain*. London: Routledge and Kegan Paul.

Jencks, C., Smith, M., Acland, H., Bane, M., Cohen, D., Gintis, H., Heyns, B. and Michelson, S. (1972) *Inequality: A Reassessment of the Effect of the Family and Schooling in America*. New York: Basic Books.

Jenkins, R. (1986) *Racism and Recruitment: Managers, Organisations and Equal Opportunity in the Labour Market*. London: Cambridge University Press.

Jenkins, R. and Troyna, B. (1983) 'Educational Myths, Labour Market Realities'. In B. Troyna and D.I. Smith (eds) *Racism, School and the Labour Market*. Leicester: National Youth Bureau.

Jones, J. (1986) *Labour of Love Labour of Sorrow: Black Women, Work and the Family, from Slavery to the Present Day*. New York: Vintage Books.

Jones, P. (1977) 'An Evaluation of the Effect of Sport on the Integration of West Indian School Children'. Unpublished Ph.D. thesis, University of Surrey.

Jordan, J. (1989) *Moving Towards Home: Political Essays*. London: Virago.

Joseph, G. (1981) 'The Incompatible Ménage à Trois: Marxism, Feminism and Racism'. In L. Sargent, *Women and Revolution*. London: Pluto Press.

Joseph, G. and Lewis, J. (1981) *Common Differences: Conflicts in Black and White Feminist Perspectives*. New York: Anchor Books.

Jules, V. (1991) 'Race and Gender as Factors of Students' Survival to the Fifth Form in Trinidad and Tobago'. In S. Ryan (ed.) *Social and Occupational Stratification in Contemporary Trinidad and Tobago*. St Augustine, Trinidad: University of the West Indies.

Junkar, P.N. (ed.) (1987) *From School to Unemployment: The Labour Market for Young People*. London: Macmillan.

Justus, J.B. (1985) 'Women's Role in West Indian Society'. In F.C. Steady (ed.) *The Black Woman Cross-culturally*. Cambridge, Mass.: Schenkman Books.

Kanter, H., Lefanu, S., Shah, S. and Spedding, C. (eds) (1984) *Sweeping Statements*. London: Women's Press.

Kearney, R. (1990) *Migration: The Irish at Home and Abroad*. Dublin: Wolfhound Press.

Khan, V.S. (1987) 'The Role of the Culture of Dominance in Structuring the Experience of Ethnic Minorities'. In C. Husband (ed.) *Race in Britain, Continuity and Change: The Second Edition*. London: Hutchinson.

King, B. (1988) 'Multiple Jeopardy, Multiple Consciousness: The Context of a Black Feminist Ideology'. *Signs*, 14 (1).

Kosack, G. (1976) 'Migrant Women: The Move to Western Europe – A Step Towards Emancipation?' *Race and Class*, 17 (4) (Spring).

Ladner, J.A. (1982) *Tomorrow's Tomorrow: The Black Women*. New York: Doubleday.

—— (1985) 'Racism and Tradition: Black Womanhood in Historical Perspective'. In F. Steady (ed.) *The Black Woman Cross-Culturally*. Cambridge, Mass.: Schenkman Books.

Lal, B.B. (1983) 'Perspectives on Ethnicity: Old Wine in New Bottles'. *Ethnic and Racial Studies*, 6 (2) (April).

Landry, B. (1987) *The New Black Middle Class*. Berkeley, Cal.: University of California Press.

Landry, B. and Jendrek, M. (1978) 'The Employment of Wives from Black Middle Class Families'. *Journal of Marriage and the Family* (Nov.).

Lashley, H. (1986) 'Prospects and Problems of Afro-Caribbeans in the British Education System'. In C. Brock (ed.) *The Caribbean in Europe: Aspects of the West Indian Experience in Britain, France and the Netherlands*. London: Frank Cass.

Lawrence, E. (1981) 'White Sociology, Black Struggle'. *Multi-Racial Education* (NAME), 9(3).

—— (1982a) 'Just Plain Common Sense: The "Roots" of Racism'. In Centre for Contemporary Cultural Studies *The Empire Strikes Back: Race and Racism in Seventies Britain*. London: Hutchinson.

—— (1982b) 'In the Abundance of Water the Fool is Thirsty: Sociology and Black "Pathology"'. In Centre for Contemporary Cultural Studies, *The Empire Strikes Back: Race and Racism in Seventies Britain*. London: Hutchinson.

Leacock, E. (1975) 'Sexual Stratification: A Cross-cultural View'. In R. Reiter (ed.) *Towards an Anthropology of Women*. New York: Monthly Review Press.

Lee, G. and Wrench, J. (1983) *Skill Seekers: Black Youth, Apprenticeships and Disadvantage*. Leicester: National Youth Bureau.

Lee, J. (1982) 'Society and Culture'. In F. Litton (ed.) *Unequal Achievement: The Irish Experience 1957–1982*. Dublin: Institute of Public Administration.

Lees, S. (1986) *Losing Out: Sexuality and Adolescent Girls*. London: Hutchinson.

Lerner, G. (ed.) (1973) *Black Women in White America: A Documentary History*. New York: Random House.

Little, A. (1975) 'The Background of Underachievement in Immigrant Children in London'. In G. Verma and C. Bagley (eds) *Race and Education Across Cultures*. London: Heinemann.

—— (1978) 'Schools and Race'. *In Five Views of Multi-Racial Britain*. London: Commission for Racial Equality.

—— (1985) 'Education for Whom?' *New Community*, 12 (2) (Summer).

Little, A., Mabey, C. and Whitaker, G. (1968) 'The Education of Immigrant Pupils in Primary Schools'. *Race*, 9 (4).

Lomas, G. (1973) *The Coloured Population of Great Britain: Census 1971*. London: Runnymede Trust.

Lomax, P. (1977) 'The Self-Concepts of Girls in the Context of a Disadvantaging Environment'. *Educational Review*, 29: 107–19.

—— (1980) 'The School Career of West Indian Immigrant Girls'. *Journal of Applied Educational Studies*, 9 (1): 29–36.

London Borough of Lambeth (1985) *Key Facts – Employment*. S. Stevens. Information Research Group, Lambeth: Directorate of Town Planning and Economic Development (May).

Louden, D. (1978) 'Self-Esteem and the Locus of Control: Some Findings on Immigrant Adolescents in Britain'. *New Community*, 7 (3): 218–34.

—— (1981) 'A Comparative Study of Self-Concepts among Minority and Majority Group Adolescents in English Multi-Racial Schools'. *Ethnic and Racial Studies*, 4 (2).

Mac an Ghaill, M. (1988) *Young, Gifted and Black: Student Teacher Relations in the Schooling of Black Youth*. Milton Keynes: Open University Press.

McAdoo, Pipes H. (ed.) (1978) 'Factors Related to Stability in Upwardly Mobile Black Families'. *Journal of Marriage and the Family* (Nov.).

—— (1988) *Black Families: 2nd edition*. London: Sage.

MacCormack, C.P. and Draper, A. (1987) 'Social and Cognitive Aspects of Female Sexuality in Jamaica'. In P. Caplan (ed.) *The Cultural Construction of Sexuality*. London: Tavistock.

MacDonald, M. (1980) 'Socio-Cultural Reproduction and Women's Education'. In R. Deem, *Schooling for Women's Work*. London: Routledge and Kegan Paul.

McDowell, D.E. (1990) 'Reading Family Matters'. In C.A. Wall (ed.) *Changing Our Own Words*. London: Routledge.

McEwan, E., Gipps, C.V. and Sumner, R. (1975) *Language Proficiency in the Multi-Racial Junior School*. Slough: NFER.

Mackintosh, N.J. and Mascie-Taylor, C.G.N. (1985) 'The IQ Question'. In DES 1985, *Education for All*, The Swann Report, HMSO, Cmnd 9453.

McRobbie, A. (1978a) 'Jackie: An Ideology of Adolescent Femininity'. Stencilled paper. Centre for Contemporary Cultural Studies, Birmingham University.

—— (1978b) 'Working Class Girls and the Culture of Femininity'. In Women's Studies Group, Centre for Contemporary Cultural Studies, *Women Take Issue*. London: Hutchinson.

—— (1980) 'Settling Accounts with Subcultures: a Feminist Critique'. *Screen Education*, 34: 37–49.

—— (1990) *Feminism and Youth Culture*. London: Macmillan Education.

McRobbie, A. and Garber, J. (1975) 'Girls and Subcultures: An Exploration'. In S. Hall and T. Jefferson (eds) *Resistance Through Rituals: Youth Subcultures in Post-war Britain*. London: Hutchinson.

Madhubuti, H.R. (1990) *Black Men: Obsolete, Single and Dangerous?* Chicago: Third World Press.

Malson, M., Mudimbe-Boyi, E., O'Barr, J. and Wyer, M. (eds) (1990) *Black Women in America: Social Science Perspectives*. Chicago: University of Chicago Press.

Mama, A. (1984) 'Black Women, the Economic Crisis and the British State'. *Feminist Review*, 17 (Autumn).

Manpower Services Commission (1981) *A New Training Initiative – An Agenda for Action*. London: MSC.

—— (1982) *Youth Task Group Report*. Moorfoot: MSC.

Manpower Services Commission/Commission for Racial Equality (1979) *Ethnic Minorities and Special Programmes for the Unemployed: The Problems, Needs and Responses*. London: MSC.

Marable, M. (1983) *How Capitalism Underdeveloped Black America: Problems in Race, Political Economy and Society*. Boston, Mass.: South End Press.

Marshall, G., Newby, H., Rose, D. and Vogler, C. (1988) *Social Class in Great Britain*. London: Hutchinson.

Massiah, J. (1982) 'Women Who Head Households'. In J. Massiah (ed.) *Women in the Caribbean, Research Papers*, Vol. 2: *Women and the Family*. Cave Hill, Barbados: Institute of Social and Economic Research, University of the West Indies.

—— (1984) 'Indicators of Women and Development: A Preliminary Framework for the Caribbean'. In J. Massiah (ed.) *Women in the Caribbean, Research Papers*, Vol. 6: *Women Work and Development*. Cave Hill, Barbados: Institute of Social and Economic Research, University of the West Indies.

—— (1986) 'Work in the Lives of Caribbean Women'. *Social and Economic Studies*. Special No.: J. Massiah (ed.) *Women in the Caribbean* (Part 1): Institute of Social and Economic Research, University of the West Indies, Vol. 35, No. 2.

—— (1988) 'Researching Women's Work: 1985 and Beyond'. In P. Mohammed and C. Shepherd *Gender in Caribbean Development*. Women and Development Studies Project, St Augustine, Trinidad: University of the West Indies.

Mathurin Mair, L. (1986) *Women Field Workers in Jamaica During Slavery: The 1986 Elsa Goveia Memorial Lecture*, Mona, Jamaica: Department of History, University of the West Indies.

Mies, M. (1983) 'Towards a Methodology for Feminist Research'. In G. Bowles and D. Klein (eds) *Theories of Women Studies*. London: Routledge and Kegan Paul.

Miles, R. (1982) *Racism and Migrant Labour*. London: Routledge.

—— (1984) 'Marxism Versus the Sociology of "Race Relations"'. *Ethnic and Racial Studies*, 7 (2), (April): 217–37.

Mills, G.W. and Mills, D.O. (1958) 'A Study of External Migration Affecting Jamaica'. *Social and Economic Studies*, 7 (2).

Milner, D. (1975) *Children and Race*. Harmondsworth: Penguin.

—— (1983) *Children and Race: Ten Years On*. London: Ward Lock Educational.

Mirza, H.S. (1984) 'Review of Janet Ward Schofield, "Black and White in School: Trust, Tension or Tolerance?"'. In *Ethnic and Racial Studies*, 7 (2) (April): 312–14.

—— (1986a) 'Absent Again? No Excuses: Black Girls and the Swann Report'. In *Ethnic and Racial Studies*, 9 (2) (April): 247–9.

—— (1986b) 'The Material Circumstances Facilitating and/or Constraining a Woman's Return to Work After the Birth of a Child'. Unpublished Report, Thomas Coram Research Unit, Institute of Education: University of London.

—— (1988) 'The Career Aspirations and Expectations of Young Black Women: The Maintenance of Inequality'. Unpublished Ph.D. thesis. University of London: Goldsmiths' College.

Mitter, S. (1988) 'Flexible Employment in the North: Dimensions of Gender and Race'. In *Women and the Economy*. The Polytechnic of North London: Women's Studies Unit.

Mohammed, P. (1982) 'Educational Attainment of Women in Trinidad and Tobago 1946–1980'. In J. Massiah (ed.) *Women in the Caribbean, Research Papers*, Vol. 5: *Women and Education*. Cave Hill, Barbados: Institute of Social and Economic Research, University of the West Indies.

—— (1988) 'The Caribbean Family Revisited'. In P. Mohammed and C. Shepherd *Gender in Caribbean Development*. Women and Development Studies Project, St Augustine, Trinidad: University of the West Indies.

Moraga, C. and Anzaldua, G. (1981) *This Bridge Called My Back: Writings by Radical Women of Color*. Watertown, Mass.: Persephone Press.

Morokvasic, M. (1983) 'Women in Migration: Beyond the Reductionist Outlook'. In A. Phizacklea (ed.) *One Way Ticket*. London: Routledge and Kegan Paul.

Mortimore, P., Sammons, P., Lewis, L. and Ecob, R. (1988) *School Matters*. London: Open Books.

Moses, Y.T. (1985) 'Female Status, the Family, and Male Dominance in a West Indian Community'. In F. Steady (ed.) *The Black Woman Cross-culturally*. Cambridge, Mass.: Schenkman Books.

Moss, P. and Brannen, J. (1988) *New Mothers at Work: Employment and Child Care*. London: Unwin Hyman.

Mullard, C. (1982) 'Multi-racial Education in Britain: From Assimilation to Cultural Pluralism'. In J. Tierney (ed.) *Race, Migration and Schooling*. Eastbourne: Holt, Rinehart & Winston.

Murray, C. (1984) *Losing Ground: America Social Policy 1950–1980*. New York: Basic Books.

—— (1990) 'Underclass'. *The Sunday Times Magazine*, (26 Nov.).

Nandy, D. (1969) 'Those Unrealistic Aspirations'. *Race Today*, 1: 166–9.

National Research Council (1989) G. Jaynes and R. Williams (eds) *A Common Destiny: Blacks and American Society*. Washington, DC.: National Academy Press.

Ngcobo, L. (1988) *Let it Be Told: Black Women Writers in Britain*. London: Virago.

Noble, J.L. (1978) *Beautiful, Also, Are the Souls of My Black Sisters*. Englewood Cliffs, NJ: Prentice-Hall.

Oakley, A. (1981) 'Interviewing Women: A Contradiction in Terms'. In H. Roberts (ed.) *Doing Feminist Research*. London: Routledge and Kegan Paul.

Office of Population and Censuses and Surveys (1980) *The Classification of Occupations and Coding Index*. OPCS, HMSO.

—— (1985) *The Labour Force Survey 1983 and 1984*. Series LFS No. 4, OPCS, HMSO.

—— (1987) *The Labour Force Survey 1985*. Series LFS No. 5, OPCS, HMSO.

Okely, J. (1987) 'Privileged, Schooled and Finished: Boarding Education for Girls'. In G. Weiner and M. Arnot (eds) *Gender Under Scrutiny*. London: Hutchinson and the Open University.

Palmer, F. (ed.) (1987) *Anti-Racism: An Assault on Education and Value*. London: Sherwood Press.

Palmer, Marynick P. (1986) 'White Women/Black Women: The Dualism of Female Identity and Experience in the United States'. In R. Takaki (ed.) *From Different Shores*. Oxford: Oxford University Press.

Parekh, B. (1983) 'Educational Opportunity in Multi-ethnic Britain'. In N. Glazer and K. Young (eds) *Ethnic Pluralism and Public Policy*. London: Heinemann.

—— (1986) 'The Politics of Multi-cultural Education in Britain'. Paper presented at the conference 'Education for All: Policies and Practices in Multi-cultural Education'. University of Manchester.

—— (1988) 'The Swann Report and Ethnic Minority Attainment'. In G. Verma and P. Pumfrey (eds) *Educational Attainments*. East Sussex: Falmer Press.

Parmar, P. (1982) 'Gender, Race and Class: Asian Women in Resistance'. In Centre for Contemporary Cultural Studies, *The Empire Strikes Back: Race and Racism in Seventies Britain*. London: Hutchinson.

—— (1989) 'Other Kinds of Dreams'. *Feminist Review*. Special issue, 'Twenty Years of Feminism', No. 31.

Parmar, P. and Mirza, N. (1981) 'Growing Angry: Growing Strong'. *Spare Rib*, 111.

Patterson, S. (1965) *Dark Strangers: A Study of West Indians in London*. Harmondsworth: Penguin.

Payne, J. (1969) 'A Comparative Study of the Mental Ability of 7- and

8-Year-Old British and West Indian Children in a West Midlands Town'. *British Journal of Educational Psychology*, 39.

Peach, C. (1968) *West Indian Migration: A Social Geography*. London: Oxford University Press.

—— (1986) 'Patterns of Afro-Caribbean Migration and Settlement in Great Britain: 1945–1981'. In C. Brock (ed.) *The Caribbean in Europe: Aspects of the West Indian Experience in Britain, France and the Netherlands*. London: Frank Cass.

Perkins, T.E. (1979) 'Rethinking Stereotypes'. In M. Barrett, P. Corrigan, A. Khun and J. Wolff (eds) *Ideology and Cultural Production*. London: Croom Helm.

Pettigrew, T.F. (1986) 'Race Relations in the USA Since 1960'. Paper presented to the Postgraduate Seminar, Goldsmiths' College, University of London.

Phillips, A. (ed.) (1987) *Feminism and Equality*. Oxford: Basil Blackwell.

Phillips, C.J. (1979) 'Educational Under-achievement in Different Ethnic Groups'. *Educational Research*, 21 (2).

Phizacklea, A. (1982) 'Migrant Women and Wage Labour: The Case of West Indian Women in Britain'. In J. West (ed.) *Work, Women and the Labour Market*. London: Routledge and Kegan Paul.

—— (1983) 'In the Front Line'. In A. Phizacklea (ed.) *One Way Ticket*. London: Routledge and Kegan Paul.

Phoenix, A. (1987) 'Theories of Gender and Black Families'. In G. Weiner and M. Arnot (eds) *Gender Under Scrutiny*. London: Hutchinson and the Open University Press.

—— (1988a) 'Narrow Definitions of Culture: The Case of Early Motherhood'. In S. Westwood and P. Bhachu (eds) *Enterprising Women: Ethnicity, Economy and Gender Relations*. London: Routledge.

—— (1988b) 'The Afro-Caribbean Myth'. *New Society* (4 March).

—— (1990) *Young Mothers?* London: Polity Press.

Pinkney, A. (1984) *The Myth of Black Progress*. Cambridge: Cambridge University Press.

Plewis, I. (1987) 'Social Disadvantage, Educational Attainment and Ethnicity: A Comment'. *British Journal of Sociology of Education*, 8: 77–82.

Powell, D. (1982) 'Network Analysis: A Suggested Model for the Study of Women and the Family in the Caribbean'. In J. Massiah (ed.) *Women in the Caribbean, Research Papers*, Vol. 2: *Women and the Family*. Cave Hill, Barbados: Institute of Social and Economic Research, University of the West Indies.

—— (1986) 'Caribbean Women and their Response to Familial Experiences', *Social and Economic Studies*, Special No. J. Massiah (ed.) *Women in the Caribbean* (Part 1): Institute of Social and Economic Research, University of the West Indies, Vol. 35, No. 2.

Prescod-Roberts, M. (1980) 'Bringing it All Back Home'. In M. Prescod-Roberts and N. Steele (eds) *Black Women: Bringing it All Back Home*. Bristol: Falling Wall Press.

Pryce, K. (1979) *Endless Pressure*. Harmondsworth: Penguin.

Race and Class (1983) 'British Racism: The Road to 1984'. Vol. 25, No. 2 (Autumn).

Rainwater, L. and Yancey, W.L. (1967) *The Moynihan Report and the Politics of Controversy*. Cambridge, Mass.: The MIT Press.

Ramazanoglu, C. (1989) *Feminism and the Contradictions of Oppression*. London: Routledge.

Ramazanoglu, C., Kazi, H., Lees, S. and Mirza, H.S. (1986) 'Feedback: Feminism and Racism'. *Feminist Review*, 22 (Spring).

Ramdin, R. (1987) *The Making of the Black Working Class in Britain*. Aldershot: Wildwood House.

Ratcliffe, P. (1988) 'Race, Class and Residence: Afro-Caribbean Households in Britain'. In C. Brock (ed.) *The Caribbean in Europe: Aspects of the West Indian Experience in Britain, France and the Netherlands*. London: Frank Cass.

Rauta, I. and Hunt, A. (1975) *Fifth Form Girls: Their Hopes for the Future*. London: HMSO.

Reddock, R. (1988) 'Feminism and Feminist Thought: An Historical Overview'. In P. Mohammed and C. Shepherd *Gender in Caribbean Development*. Women and Development Studies Project, St Augustine, Trinidad: University of the West Indies.

Redfern, B. (1989) *Women of Color in the US: A Guide to the Literature*. New York: Garland.

Reid, E. (1989) 'Black Girls Talking'. *Gender and Education*: Special Issue: 'Race, Gender and Education' O. Foster-Carter and C. Wright (eds), Vol. 1, No. 3.

Rex, J. (1988) *The Ghetto and the Underclass: Essays on Race and Social Policy*. Aldershot: Avebury Gower Publishing.

Rex, J. and Tomlinson, S. (1979) *Colonial Immigrants in a British City*. London: Routledge.

Rex, J. and Mason, D. (eds) (1988) *Theories of Race and Ethnic Relations*. Cambridge: Cambridge University Press.

Rhodes, E. and Braham, P. (1987) 'Equal Opportunity in the Context of High Levels of Unemployment'. In R. Jenkins and J. Solomos (eds) *Racism and Equal Opportunity Policies in the 1980s*. Cambridge: Cambridge University Press.

Rich, A. (1976) 'Women's Studies – Renaissance or Revolution?' *Women's Studies*, 3 (2).

Riessman, C. (1987) 'When Gender Is Not Enough: Interviewing Women Interviewing Women'. *Gender and Society*, 1 (2).

Riley, K. (1985) 'Black Girls Speak for Themselves'. In G. Weiner (ed.) *Just a Bunch of Girls*. Milton Keynes: Open University Press.

Rist, R. (1970) 'Student Social Class and Teacher Expectations: The Self-fulfilling Prophecy in Ghetto Education'. *Harvard Educational Review*, 40 (Aug.): 411–50.

Roberts, H. (1983) 'Boys will be Boys – But What Happens to the Girls?' *Educational Research*, 25 (2).

—— (1987) 'The Social Classification of Women: A Life-cycle Approach'. In P. Allatt, T. Keil, A. Bryman and B. Bytheway (eds) *Women and the Life-cycle Approach*. London: Macmillan.

Roberts, K. (1984) *School Leavers and Their Prospects: Youth and the Labour Market in the 1980s*. Milton Keynes: Open University Press.

Roberts, K., Duggan, J. and Noble, M. (1983a) 'Young, Black and Out of Work'. In B. Troyna and D.I. Smith (eds) *Racism, School and the Labour Market*. Leicester: National Youth Bureau.

—— (1983b) 'Racial Disadvantage in the Youth Labour Market'. In L. Barton and S. Walker (eds) *Race, Class and Education*. Beckenham, Kent: Croom Helm.

Rodgers-Rose, L.F. (ed.) (1980) *The Black Woman*. Beverly Hills, Cal.: Sage Publications.

Rollins, J. (1985) *Between Women: Domestics and their Employers*. Philadelphia, Pa.: Temple University Press.

Rose, E.J.B. *et al.* (1969) *Colour and Citizenship: A Report on British Race Relations*. London: Oxford University Press.

Rosen, H. and Burgess, T. (1980) *Language and Dialects of London School Children: An Investigation*. London: Ward Lock Educational.

Rosenberg, M. and Simmons, G. (1972) *Black and White Self-esteem: The Urban School Child*. Washington, DC: American Sociological Association, Rose Monograph.

Rubovits, P. and Maehr, M. (1973) 'Pygmalion Black and White'. *Journal of Personality and Social Psychology*, 25: 210–18.

Runnymede Trust (1989) *Racism, Anti-racism and Schools: A Summary of the Burnage Report*. London: Runnymede Trust.

Runnymede Trust and Radical Statistics Race Group (1980) *Britain's Black Population*. London: Heinemann.

Rutter, M. (1981) *Maternal Deprivation Reassessed*. Harmondsworth: Penguin.

Rutter, M., Gray, G., Maughan, B. and Smith, A. (1982) 'School Experiences and the First Year of Employment'. Unpublished Report to the DES.

Rutter, M., Maughan, B., Mortimore, P. and Ouston, J. (1979) *Fifteen Thousand Hours*. London: Open Books.

Ryan, C. (1987) 'London Irish'. *New Society* (30 Jan.).

Ryan, W. (1967) 'Savage Discovery: *The Moynihan Report*'. In L. Rainwater and W. Yancey *The Moynihan Report and the Politics of Controversy*. Cambridge, Mass.: The MIT Press.

—— (1971) *Blaming the Victim*. New York: Random House.

Sage: A Scholarly Journal on Black Women (April 1984), Special issue: 'Black Women in Education'.

Saint Victor, R. (1986) 'Family Relations and Support Systems'. In P. Ellis (ed.) *Women of the Caribbean*. London: Zed Books.

Sarup, M. (1986) *The Politics of Multi-racial Education*. London: Routledge and Kegan Paul.

Sassen-Koob, S. (1984) 'From Household to Work Place: Theories and Survey Research on Migrant Women in the Labour Market'. *International Migration Review*, 18 (4).

Schlegel, A. (ed.) (1977) *Sexual Stratification: A Cross-cultural View*. New York.

Schofield, J.W. (1982) *Black and White in School: Trust, Tension or Tolerance*, New York: Praeger.

Schools Council (1972) *Careers Education in the 1970s*. Working paper no. 40. London: Evans Bros.

Scott, P.B. (1982) 'Debunking Sapphire: Towards a Non-Racist and Non-Sexist Social Science'. In G.T. Hull, P.B. Scott and B. Smith (eds) *All the Women Are White, All the Blacks Are Men, But Some of Us Are Brave*. New York: The Feminist Press.

Segal, L. (1987) *Is the Future Female?* London: Virago.

—— (1990) *Slow Motion: Changing Masculinities, Changing Men*. London: Virago.

Sewell, W.H. and Shah, V.P. (1977) 'Socio-economic Status, Intelligence, and the Attainment of Higher Education'. In J. Karabel and A.H. Halsey (eds) *Power and Ideology in Education*. New York: Oxford University Press.

Shacklady Smith, L. (1978) 'Sexist Assumptions and Female Delinquency'. In C. Smart and B. Smart, *Women, Sexuality and Social Control*. London: Routledge and Kegan Paul.

Shah, S. (1989) 'Effective Permeation of Race and Gender Issues in Teacher Education Courses'. *Gender and Education*, Special issue, 'Race and Education' O. Foster-Carter and C. Wright (eds) , Vol. 1, No. 3.

—— (1990) 'Equal Opportunity Issues in the Context of the National Curriculum: A Black Perspective', *Gender and Education*, 2 (3).

Sharp, R. and Green, A. (1976) *Education and Social Control*. London: Routledge and Kegan Paul.

Sharpe, S. (1987; 1st edn, 1976) *Just Like a Girl: How Girls Learn to be Women*. Harmondsworth: Penguin.

Shorey-Bryan, N. (1986) 'The Making of Male–Female Relationships in the Caribbean'. In P. Ellis (ed.) *Women of the Caribbean*. London: Zed Books.

Sillitoe, K. and Meltzer, H. (1985) *The West Indian School Leaver:* Vol. 1, *Starting Work*. OPCS, Social Survey Division: HMSO.

Simms, M. (1988) 'The Choices that Young Black Women Make: Education, Employment, and Family Formation'. Working paper no. 190, Wellesley College Center for Research on Women. Wellesley, Mass.

Simms, M. and Malveaux, J. (eds) (1986) *Slipping Through the Cracks: The Status of Black Women*. New Brunswick, NJ: Transaction Books.

Sivanandan, A. (1976) 'Race, Class and the State: The Black Experience in Britain'. *Race and Class*, 17 (4) (Spring).

—— (1982) *A Different Hunger*. London: Pluto Press.

—— (1990) *Communities in Resistance: Writings on Black Struggles for Socialism*. London: Verso.

Smith, D. (1977) *Racial Disadvantage in Britain*. Harmondsworth: Pelican.

Smith, D. and Tomlinson, S. (1989) *The School Effect: A Study of Multi-racial Comprehensives*. London: PSI.

Smith, M.G. (1962) *West Indian Family Structure*. Seattle, Wash.: University of Washington Press.

Smith, S. (1989) *The Politics of Race and Residence*. London: Polity Press.

Solomos, J. (1986) 'The Social and Political Context of Black Youth Unemployment: A Decade of Policy Developments and the Limits of Reform'. In L. Barton and S. Walker (eds) *Youth, Unemployment and Schooling*. Milton Keynes: Open University Press.

Spelman, E.V. (1988) *Inessential Woman: Problems of Exclusion in Feminist Thought*. Boston: Beacon Press.

Spender, D. and Sarah, E. (eds) (1980) *Learning to Lose: Sexism in Education*. London: The Women's Press.

Spillers, H. (1990) 'The Permanent Obliquity of an In(pha)llibly Straight: In the Time of Daughters and Fathers'. In C.A. Wall. *Changing Our Own Words*. London: Routledge.

Stack, C.B. (1974) *All Our Kin: Strategies for Survival in a Black Community*. New York: Harper & Row.

—— (1985) 'Sex Roles and Survival Strategies in the Urban Black Community'. In F.C. Steady (ed.) *The Black Woman Cross-Culturally*. Cambridge, Mass.: Schenkman Books.

Stanley, L. and Wise, S. (1983) *Breaking Out: Feminist Consciousness and Feminist Research*. London: Routledge and Kegan Paul.

Stanworth, M. (1977) *Gender and Schooling: A Study of Sexual Divisions in the Classroom*. London: Hutchinson in association with Explorations in Feminism Collective.

Staples, R. (1985a) 'Changes in Black Family Structure: The Conflict Between Family Ideology and Structural Conditions'. *Journal of Marriage and the Family*, 47: 1005–13.

—— (1985b) 'The Myth of Matriarchy'. In F.C. Steady (ed.) *The Black Woman Cross-culturally*. Cambridge, Mass.: Schenkman Books.

—— (1986: 1st edition, 1982) *Black Masculinity*. San Francisco: Black Scholar Press.

Steady, F. (1985; 1st edition, 1981) *The Black Woman Cross-culturally*. Cambridge, Mass.: Schenkman Books.

Stone, J. (1985) *Racial Conflict in Contemporary Society*. London: Fontana and William Collins.

Stone, K. (1983) 'Motherhood and Waged Work: West Indian, Asian and White Mothers Compared'. In A. Phizacklea (ed.) *One Way Ticket*. London: Routledge and Kegan Paul.

Stone, M. (1985: 1st edition, 1981) *The Education of the Black Child: The Myth of Multi-cultural Education*. London: Fontana Press.

Sutton, C. and Makiesky-Barrow, S. (1977) 'Social Inequality and Sexual Status in Barbados'. In A. Schlegel (ed.) *Sexual Stratification: A Cross-cultural View*. New York: Columbia University Press.

Tang Nain, G. (1991) 'Black Women, Sexism and Racism: Black or Antiracist Feminism?' *Feminist Review*, 37 (Spring).

Taylor, M.J. (1981) *Caught Between: A Review of Research into the Education of Pupils of West Indian Origin*. Slough: NFER.

Thomas-Hope, E. (1986) 'Caribbean Diaspora – The Inheritance of Slavery: Migration from the Commonwealth Caribbean'. In C. Brock (ed.) *The Caribbean in Europe: Aspects of the West Indian Experience in Britain, France and the Netherlands*. London: Frank Cass.

Thorogood, N. (1987) 'Race, Class and Gender: The Politics of Housework'. In J. Brannen and G. Wilson (eds) *Give and Take in Families*. London: Allen & Unwin.

Tidrick, G. (1973) 'Some Aspects of Jamaican Emigration to the United Kingdom 1953–1962'. In L. Comitas and D. Lowenthal (eds) *Work and Family Life: West Indian Perspectives*. New York: Anchor Books.

Timberlake, A., Weber Cannon, L., Guy, R. and Higginbotham, E. (1988) *Women of Color and Southern Women: A Bibliography of Social Science Research: 1975–1988*. Memphis, Tenn.: Memphis State University Center for Research on Women.

Tizard, B., Blatchford, P., Burke, J., Farquhar, C., and Plewis, I. (1988) *Young Children at School in the Inner City*. London: Lawrence, Erlbaum Associates.

Tomlinson, S. (1981) *Educational Subnormality: A Study in Decision Making*. London: Routledge and Kegan Paul.

—— (1982) 'Response of the English Education System to the Children of Immigrant Parentage'. M. Leggon (ed.) *Research in Racial and Ethnic Relations*, Vol. 3.

—— (1983a) *Ethnic Minorities in British Schools: A Review of the Literature, 1960–82*. London: Heinemann Educational Books.

—— (1983b) 'Black Women in Higher Education – Case Studies of University Women in Britain'. In L. Barton and S. Walker (eds) *Race, Class and Education*. Beckenham, Kent: Croom Helm.

—— (1985) 'The "Black Education" Movement'. In M. Arnot (ed.) *Race and Gender*. Oxford: Pergamon Press in association with the Open University.

—— (1987) 'Towards AD 2000: The Political Context of Multi-cultural Education'. *New Community*, XIV (1/2) (Autumn).

—— (1990) 'Effective Schooling for Ethnic Minorities', *New Community*, 16 (3).

Troyna, B. (ed.) (1987) *Racial Inequality in Education*. London: Tavistock.

—— (1988) 'British Schooling and the Reproduction of Racial Inequality'. In C. Brock (ed.) *The Caribbean in Europe: Aspects of the West Indian Experience in Britain, France and the Netherlands*. London: Frank Cass.

—— (1990) 'Reform or Deform? The 1988 Education Reform Act and

Racial Inequality in Britain', *New Community*, 16 (3).

Troyna, B. and Ball, W. (1985) 'Educational Decision Making and Issues of Race'. In *The Quarterly Journal of Social Affairs*, 4 (1).

Troyna, B. and Williams, J. (1986) *Racism, Education and the State*. London: Croom Helm.

Ullah, P. (1985a) 'Disaffected Black and White Youth: The Role of Unemployment Duration and Perceived Job Discrimination'. *Ethnic and Racial Studies*. 8 (2) (April).

—— (1985b) 'Second-Generation Irish Youth: Identity and Ethnicity'. *New Community*. XII (2) (Summer).

VanDyke, R.M. (1985) 'Secondary School Careers Advice, Examination Choices and Adult Aspirations: The Maintenance of Gender Stratification'. Unpublished PhD London School of Economics and Political Science. University of London.

Veness, T. (1962) *School Leavers*. London: Methuen.

Verma, G.K. With Ashworth, B. (1986) *Ethnicity and Educational Achievement in British Schools*. London: Macmillan Press.

Walker, A. (1983) *In Search of Our Mothers' Gardens*. New York: Harcourt Brace and Jovanovich.

Wall, C.A. (ed.) (1990) *Changing Our Own Words: Essays on Criticism, Theory, and Writing by Black Women*. London: Routledge.

Wallace, C. (1987) *For Richer for Poorer: Growing Up In and Out of Work*. London: Tavistock.

Wallace, M. (1979) *Black Macho and the Myth of the Superwoman*. London: Calder.

—— (1982) 'A Black Feminist's Search for Sisterhood'. In G.T. Hull, P.B. Scott and B. Smith (eds) *All the Women Are White, All the Blacks Are Men, But Some of Us Are Brave*. New York: The Feminist Press.

Ware, V. (1991) *Beyond the Pale: White Women, Racism and History*. London: Verso.

Washington, M.H. (1984) 'I Sign my Mother's Name: Alice Walker, Dorothy West, Paule Marshall'. In R. Perry and M. Watson Brownley (eds) *Mothering the Mind*. New York: Holmes and Meier.

—— (1989) *Invented Lives: Narratives of Black Women 1860–1960*. London: Virago.

Weinreich, P. (1979) 'Cross-Ethnic Identification and Self-Rejection in a Black Adolescent'. In G.K. Verma and C. Bagley (eds) *Race, Education and Identity*, London: Macmillan.

Westwood, S. and Bhachu, P. (1988) *Enterprising Women: Ethnicity, Economy, and Gender Relations*. London: Routledge.

Wilkie, J.R. (1985) 'The Decline of Occupational Segregation Between Black and White Women'. *Research in Ethnic and Racial Relations*, 4.

Williams, J. (1985) 'Redefining Institutional Racism'. *Ethnic and Racial Studies*, 8 (3).

Williams, M. (1986) 'The Thatcher Generation'. *New Society* (21 Feb.).

Willis, P. (1977) *Learning to Labour: How Working Class Kids Get Working Class Jobs.* Farnborough: Saxon House.

—— (1979) 'Shop Floor Culture, Masculinity and the Wage Form'. In J. Clarke, C. Critcher and R. Johnson (eds) *Working Class Culture.* London: Hutchinson in association with the Centre for Contemporary Cultural Studies, Birmingham.

—— (1983) 'The Class Significance of School Counter-Culture'. In J. Purvis and M. Hales (eds) *Achievement and Inequality in Education.* London: Routledge and Kegan Paul.

Willis, S. (1987) *Specifying: Black American Women Writing the American Experience.* Madison, Wis.: University of Wisconsin Press.

Wilson, P. (1969) 'Reputation and Respectability: A Suggestion for Caribbean Ethnology'. *Man* (no. 3) 4 (1).

Wilson, W.J. (1978) *The Declining Significance of Race.* Chicago: University of Chicago Press.

—— (1987) *The Truly Disadvantaged: The Inner City, the Under Class, and Public Policy.* Chicago: University of Chicago Press.

Wiltshire-Brodber, R. (1988) 'Gender, Race and Class in the Caribbean'. In P. Mohammed and C. Shepherd *Gender in Caribbean Development.* Women and Development Studies Project, St Augustine, Trinidad: University of the West Indies.

Wrench, J. (1990) 'New Vocationalism, Old Racism and the Careers Service'. *New Community,* 16 (3).

Wright, C. (1987) 'The Relations Between Teachers and Afro-Caribbean Pupils: Observing Multi-racial Classrooms'. In G. Weiner and M. Arnot (eds) *Gender Under Scrutiny.* London: Hutchinson in association with the Open University.

Wulff, H. (1988) *Twenty Girls: Growing Up, Ethnicity and Excitement in a South London Microculture.* Stockholm Studies in Anthropology, 21. Stockholm: University of Stockholm.

Yekwai, D. (1986) *British Racism, Miseducation and the Afrikan Child.* London: Karnak House.

Yule, W., Berger, M., Rutter, M. and Yule, B. (1975) 'Children of West Indian Immigrants, Intellectual Performance and Reading Attainment'. *Journal of Child Psychology and Psychiatry,* 16.

Name index

Subject index

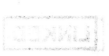

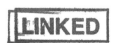